The Essentia~ ~f Com~~ ~ty Care

2nd editio~

Also by Peter Sharkey

Introducing Community Care

The Essentials of Community Care

Second edition

Peter Sharkey

Consultant Editor: Jo Campling

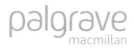

First published 2007 by
PALGRAVE MACMILLAN
Houndmills, Basingstoke, Hampshire RG21 6XS and
175 Fifth Avenue, New York, N.Y. 10010
Companies and representatives throughout the world

PALGRAVE MACMILLAN is the global academic imprint of the Palgrave Macmillan division of St. Martin's Press, LLC and of Palgrave Macmillan Ltd. Macmillan® is a registered trademark in the United States, United Kingdom and other countries. Palgrave is a registered trademark in the European Union and other countries.

ISBN-13: 978–1–4039–4203–6
ISBN-10: 1–4039–4203–X

This book is printed on paper suitable for recycling and made from fully managed and sustained forest sources. Logging, pulping and manufacturing processes are expected to conform to the environmental regulations of the country of origin.

A catalogue record for this book is available from the British Library.

10   9   8   7   6   5   4   3   2
16   15   14   13   12   11   10   09   08   07

Printed in China

To Cindy, Kieran and Sarah

Contents

List of Figures

Introduction

This is a book primarily for students preparing to be social care and health-care practitioners. It is also a book for current practitioners of social care and healthcare, for social policy students interested in community care and for anyone wanting an introductory overview of the main issues in community care. This second edition updates the first edition that was published in 2000.

Since the first edition there have been a number of changes in policy and practice and this edition hopes to capture the main elements of these by updating and modifying each chapter. On a personal level, I have left full-time work in higher education and returned to part-time social work practice with older people as well as becoming an Associate Lecturer with the Open University on the course 'Care, Welfare and Community' (course K202). Both sets of experiences have had some influence on the contents of this second edition. Since my return to practice, I have worked in three social work situations. People often ask, 'What is it like?' My usual answer is that the issues and problems that people in the community face are much the same but that the ways of approaching them and dealing with them have certainly changed a lot. Some interesting and exciting changes have taken place. To pick out a few – there is much more flexible community provision, enabling people to stay in the community; there is more thought given to providing supportive housing situations; 'direct payments' are now available for different user groups, enabling different forms of support and care; there is a strong emphasis on listening to and involving service users; and there is a strong emphasis on practitioners working together to provide 'integrated care'. I hope that the book will capture some of the changes and some of the problems and possibilities for practitioners.

Community care is a fascinating area of study, raising important questions about how we organise and care for the most vulnerable members of society, who should do that caring and who should pay for it. Underpinning discussions of community care are important questions of values, such as how much do we care for those adults in society who are most vulnerable and in what way should we care for them?

Community care is usually seen as being about social care and support for people in the community. However, health provision is a major dimension of any care within the community. Hence, in this book the term 'practitioners' is often used as a generic term to describe community nurses, community occupational therapists, social workers and other professional workers involved in community care.

The present community care system, which developed during the early 1990s, was formulated when the government philosophy in relation to health and social care was one of expanding the role of the market. Those who supported this policy (and the wider expansion of the role of the market throughout society) were often called the 'New Right', and the changes in community care need to be understood within this wider context. New Right policies led to a curtailing of the powers of local authorities, a focus on the development of a competitive market, the development of a strong individualistic ethos and the targeting of individuals for provision and help.

One problem with this general approach is that its focus on individual problems has neglected the wider context. Practitioners and managers often feel bombarded by individual problems and demands. It can sometimes seem hard to see the wider connections because of these often relentless pressures. However, individuals need to be seen within the wider societal structures within which they are found. There are links to be made, for example, between poverty and mental health. We shall see that the policies of the late 1980s and the 1990s individualised community care issues by emphasising individual packages of care and eligibility criteria. The targeting of particular people with problems has played a part in divorcing community care from the communities and societal structures within which it takes place. This book will try to make connections with the wider picture. While the election of the Labour government in 1997 continued many of the 'market' policies of its predecessor, it did at least acknowledge the links between, for example, health and inequality (DoH, 1999b) and proposed policies to deal with social exclusion.

The current community care system is embedded in the National Health Service and Community Care Act 1990. Discussion of this Act is central to this book and the abbreviation NHS&CC Act 1990 is used throughout. The Act applied to all parts of the United Kingdom and therefore the community care systems of Scotland, Wales, Northern Ireland and England share many common features. However, there are differences, especially since devolution came into effect in 1999, and some of these differences are indicated in the text.

A book entitled *The Essentials of Community Care* involves some selection and some judgement about what the 'essentials' are. The issues chosen are those in which a sound knowledge of the background context is important if practitioners are to develop good, reflective practice. Personal beliefs have also influenced the content. My personal view is that community care developments have been too focused on providing individual solutions rather than addressing community issues and wider structural issues. I believe a more critical perspective needs to be given to the role of private business in health and social care provision. I also believe that more attention needs to be given to the relationship between practitioners and unpaid carers within the community.

Chapter 1 outlines the background to the NHS&CC Act 1990, the changes it introduced to community care and the subsequent developments during the 1990s. Most community care is provided by relatives, neighbours and friends and Chapter 2 focuses on this aspect of care in the community. A key question during the 1990s and into the new century has been 'who should provide what'? There have been particular tensions about and changes to the boundaries of health and social care provision. Chapter 3 outlines the background to this and the way in which the boundaries of community care provision have been shifting, using the long-term care of older people as an illustration. Probably the most significant change for practitioners after the passage of the NHS&CC Act 1990, was the introduction of care management, and this is the concern of Chapter 4. A variety of professional workers are involved in the delivery of community care provision and a central problem is the structures under which they have to work. These structures have often impeded their ability to work together, and this is the theme of Chapter 5. This links into the topic of the relationship between professional workers and informal care networks, which is central to the discussion in Chapter 6. Chapter 7 examines user empowerment and some of the changes and development in this area. Child abuse has been a major concern of social and healthcare professionals for many years but the abuse of adults has not been given similar attention and concern. This is changing and Chapter 8 examines aspects of the abuse of adults within the context of community care.

Some of the overarching themes of the book that cut across different chapters and help to integrate the material are:

- Boundary problems between agencies.
- The importance of working constructively with other practitioners.
- Seeing 'individuals' within the wider structural context of their situation.
- Acknowledgement of diversity and the need for anti-oppressive practice to respond to this.

- The importance of service-user involvement and empowerment.
- The continuing tensions in health and social care between promoting independence and exercising some protection of adults in vulnerable situations.
- Working with and alongside carers and the community in relation to community care.
- The increasing role of private businesses in providing aspects of health and social care.

A summary of the subject matter to be covered is provided at the beginning of each chapter. In many chapters, practice issues are threaded through the material, but all of the chapters end with a section on issues of concern and relevance to practitioners, followed by some further reading for those who wish to follow up a topic. Where helpful, a suggestion of pertinent World Wide Web sites is also provided. Community care is a moving picture and the web sites help readers to keep up-to-date with developments. Their exploration should be seen as an important element of learning about community care and keeping up to date with changes. Unless otherwise stated, the case studies used are fictitious but they are intended to resemble typical real situations.

Terminology varies across professional groupings. In this book 'service user' is generally used to describe people who use community care services. While perhaps not an ideal description, I hope it is acceptable to the various professional groups and to service users themselves. In other areas of description, an effort has been made to avoid terminology that might be seen as offensive or oppressive, and it is hoped that this has been achieved. Local authority departments with responsibilities for adults have different names in different areas. For example, they might be called Adult Social Care Services or Community Care Services. The term 'social service authorities' is used to describe these.

Past and present colleagues and students have helped in various ways in relation to the book. I cannot name them all and am grateful to them for their help and support. Jo Campling and staff at Palgrave have been a ready source of advice and help on the publishing side. Thanks also to Palgrave's external reviewers for helpful comments. Cindy Sharkey has read drafts, made corrections and offered ideas – thus making a substantial contribution to the process of preparing both editions. Thanks, as ever, to her.

Peter Sharkey

CHAPTER 1

Background to Community Care

Chapter summary

This chapter covers:

- The background to and community care content of the NHS&CC Act 1990.
- Key aspects of what the government was trying to do in relation to community care.
- How local authorities responded to the financial pressures upon them.
- The need to connect individual community care concerns to wider issues of public policy and structural inequality.

Introduction

Community care is hard to define. One broad understanding is the care of people within the community who have previously lived in long-stay institutions. A second element focuses on efforts to keep disabled people, older people and vulnerable people within the community rather than seeing them having to go into institutional care. A third key issue is the considerable unpaid support and help given by relatives, friends and neighbours.

In terms of those who receive care, it is possible to take a narrow definition of community care and see it as essentially the care within the community of older people, people with learning difficulties, people with physical disabilities and people with mental health problems. However, a wider definition would include several other groups, for example:

- People with a sensory impairment.
- People with problems arising from the use of drugs or alcohol.
- Victims of domestic violence.
- Homeless people.
- Vulnerable single parents.

- People with HIV/AIDS.
- Ex-offenders.
- Asylum-seekers and refugees.
- People requiring palliative care.
- People now in the community after many years in hospital.

The great majority of community care is provided by informal carers, usually family members (explored in detail in Chapter 2). This means that most of us have some personal experience of aspects of community care. These experiences can often open our eyes to the complexities and stresses of caring and issues concerning the services available. One personal experience is described in Box 1.1.

Box 1.1   A personal experience

In *Remind Me Who I Am, Again*, Linda Grant (1999) describes the life of her Jewish mother, especially during her later years, when she was disabled by dementia. In the book there are many insights into the disease, the dilemmas and emotions of caring, and the community care system. Grant was motivated to write the book 'Because there is a silence, a taboo. No one knows how to feel, or what to think because the meteor of dementia that strikes families and wipes out so much is supposed to be part of the realm of privacy. What you don't talk about. What you keep to yourself' (ibid., 1999, p. 300). Grant and others have begun to break the taboo of silence and provide us with powerful prose on the experiences and feelings involved. Many of us will experience something similar in our own personal lives.

Aspects of community care are quite commonly headlined in the media. Social workers may be blamed for 'bed-blocking' in hospitals through delays in assessment, an old person may die of abuse or neglect, or mental health services may be claimed to be in disarray following some incident. These are 'human interest' stories because they could relate so easily to ourselves, our family or our friends.

This chapter sets the scene for the later chapters by covering the changes in community care services since 1990. It outlines what governments have tried to achieve and how agencies have responded. After the passage of the postwar welfare state legislation, with its background in the Beveridge Report, there were several white papers and reports on aspects of community care but little actual legislation. It is for this reason that the NHS&CC Act 1990 stands out as a major piece of legislation in the postwar period.

Various postwar governments made some effort to develop community care policies, but these were not pursued with great energy or determination and by the mid 1980s most commentators and politicians of all political parties agreed that a lot was wrong with community care.

The social care changes

The Audit Commission's *Making a Reality of Community Care* (1986) was very critical of community care as it was operating. The report stressed the need for some urgent reform of the financing and organising of community care, 'The one option that is not tenable is to do nothing about present financial, organisational and staffing arrangements' (ibid., p. 4). Central to its critique was the existence of 'perverse incentives' (Department of Social Security funding) for care to be provided in residential and nursing homes but a lack of comparable funds to help those who preferred to remain in their own homes.

The government responded to the Audit Commission's Report by commissioning a further report from Roy Griffiths. One of the key recommendations of the Griffiths Report (1988) was that the lead authority in relation to community care should be the local authority. This recommendation was not initially popular with a government that had tried to curb the power and influence of local authorities over the preceding years. There was more than a year's delay before the government responded. A range of possible alternative ways of organising community care were apparently looked at before falling back on Griffiths' idea of local authority responsibility.

Most of Griffiths' recommendations found their way into the important White Paper *Caring for People* (DoH, 1989a). The White Paper contained two separate chapters on community care in Wales and Scotland. There was a separate White Paper for Northern Ireland (DHSS, 1990), reflecting the very different administrative arrangements there. Shortly after the publication of *Caring for People*, the government introduced the National Health Service and Community Care Bill, which included provisions for implementing the plans set out in the White Paper. Between December 1989 and June 1990, the Bill progressed through parliament and received Royal Assent in late June 1990.

Although the community care aspects of the Act occupied only a few sections, they set the framework for community care provision over the following years. The Act was implemented in three stages during 1991–93. For example, in 1991 each social service authority had to have set up an inspection unit in relation to all residential homes. However, the big change was in relation to financing and this came in 1993 with the transfer of responsibilities and money to local social service authorities. After April 1993, prospective residents of residential and nursing homes had to approach these authorities for help with fees.

Some argue that community care law has remained in a poor shape since the 1990 Act, that it is deeply rooted in earlier legislation and that it leaves social service authorities and social workers open to litigation. Clements, for example, believes that the legislation needs to be unified and clarified and that 'Community care law remains a hotchpotch of conflicting statutes, which have been enacted over a period of 50 years; each statute reflects the different philosophical attitudes of its time' (Clements, 2004, p. 8).

Box 1.2   Beethoven and community care

Luke Clements' book *Community Care and the Law* (3rd edn, 2004) is a useful source of further information on the law. His book has a picture of Beethoven on the cover. The point is made that at some point in our lives many of us will have community care needs. Beethoven came from a troubled family and had a father with a serious drink problem. In adult life Beethoven gradually lost his hearing and was profoundly deaf in his later years. In our day he would probably be a user of community care services. Unable to hear his own compositions, at times in considerable despair, neglectful of his person and living in poor and untidy conditions he produced some of the most wonderful music that the world has heard.

As the 1990s progressed, some of the weaknesses of the 1990 community care legislation became clearer. For example, it neglected carers, failed adequately to promote independent living and did not address the abuse of vulnerable adults. Some of the faults were addressed by piecemeal legislation such as that on carers (Carers Recognition and Services Act 1995) and independent living (Community Care (Direct Payments) Act 1996). Chapter 8 covers the way in which the issue of adult abuse has been addressed since 1990.

In late 1998, a new White Paper for England was published, entitled *Modernising Social Services* (DoH, 1998a). This outlined the new Labour government's future plans for social care and White Papers with a largely similar content were published shortly afterwards for Northern Ireland, Scotland and Wales. There were no dramatic changes, rather the emphasis was on improving the existing facilities, or modernising rather than restructuring them. However Labour put greater emphasis on promoting independence, providing services more consistently across the country and making the system more centred on service users. Several new initiatives were intended to contribute towards these objectives including an emphasis on prevention and rehabilitation, a National Carers' Strategy, National Service Frameworks for user groups, guidance on Fair Access to Care and Better Government for Older People (ibid.). Labour also appointed a Royal Commission on Long Term Care, which reported early in 1999 (Sutherland, 1999).

The theme of 'modernisation' ran through all of the policy documents and the changes. Another significant theme was the importance of organisations working together in 'partnership' and breaking down the traditional divisions between health care and social care (this is discussed further in Chapters 3 and 5). The concern with human rights, reflected in the passage of the Human Rights Act 1998 (see Box 1.3), also had an impact on community care practice.

Box 1.3   The Human Rights Act 1998 and community care

The Human Rights Act 1998 was implemented in October 2000. It applied across the United Kingdom and it made the European Convention on Human Rights part of UK law. It was intended that the philosophy of human rights should become part of the UK legal systems and of UK culture and this included the whole area of community care. Organisations have the duty to uphold rights scheduled in the Act's articles. The most relevant sections of the convention to community care are:
Article 2: Right to life.
Article 3: Right not to be subjected to inhuman or degrading treatment.
Article 5: Right not to be arbitrarily deprived of liberty.
Article 6: Right to a fair hearing.
Article 8: Right to respect for private and family life.
Article 14: Right not to be discriminated against.

Variations within the United Kingdom

The previous section has made reference to the different countries of the United Kingdom and how community care was dealt with in the White Papers of 1989 and 1998. The NHS&CC Act 1990 applied to all parts of the United Kingdom. Prior to 1999, Wales and England had had a shared legal system and community care developments in the two countries were similar. In Scotland, a similar system of provision and procedures evolved in the early years after the 1990 Act (Petch *et al.*, 1996). Some writers have noted that developments on the ground were perhaps slower in Scotland than elsewhere (Douglas and Philpott, 1998). Northern Ireland had had a very different administrative structure as a result of direct rule in the province. With the introduction of direct rule, an alternative had to be found to local government welfare provision. The pragmatic solution was to link this to the health service structure. This resulted in a unified health and social services structure under the auspices of four boards, set up in 1973 and accountable to Westminster through the Northern Ireland civil service and the Secretary of State. The board members were directly appointed by ministers.

Part of the manifesto pledge of the incoming 1997 Labour government was a commitment to devolution. The new Scottish Parliament and Welsh Assembly met for the first time in 1999. Likewise, in Northern Ireland, following the 'Good Friday Agreement' (1998), a Northern Ireland Assembly and Executive was introduced in 1999. This has operated for periods and reverted to 'direct rule' for periods since then. Thus from 1999, Scotland, Wales and Northern Ireland all had an independent parliament or national assembly with certain devolved powers from the Westminster government. In relation to community care, somewhat different organisational structures and regulatory systems have been set up leading to some variation in provision. Chapter 3 outlines how personal care is now paid for by the state in Scotland but not elsewhere in United Kingdom. Scotland also was the first country to implement new legislation relating to decision-making capacity with the Adults with Incapacity (Scotland) Act 2000. A further example of variation is that England has been the only country to introduce a fining system for delayed discharge from hospitals and it did this in 2004.

As a result of these developments, the reader should bear in mind throughout the book that there is some variation between parts of the United Kingdom and further research may well be needed for a particular country. Web sites mentioned at the end of this chapter will help to facilitate this exploration and readers are encouraged to explore the appropriate sections of these sites. However, over many areas the principles and practice of community care do remain similar throughout the United Kingdom.

Key objectives of government policies

In relation to community care, the 1990 legislation contained a number of key policy objectives and the main ones are summarised below.

Control on expenditure

In the 1970s, supplementary benefits were administered in a way that gave considerable discretion to social security officers and local offices. One aspect of this was assisting residents of private residential or nursing homes who found themselves in financial difficulty. In 1979, only £10 million was spent in this way. From 1980, the rules under which people could claim board and lodging expenses were regulated by parliamentary statute and residents or boarders could claim full board and lodging plus an amount to cover personal expenses. Local authorities under financial pressure need no longer build new residential homes, and health authorities could close long-stay wards without appearing heartless. As Lewis and Glennerster (1996, p. 4) wrote, 'In short, the social security budget had come to the rescue of families, local authorities, and the NHS, all of them under tight budgetary limits and increasing demand'.

During the 1980s, there was a rapid rise in social security payments to people in residential and nursing homes from £10 million in 1979 to £2,600 million in 1993 (Richards, 1996, p. 9). Concern about the exponential growth of this expenditure was reflected in various reports and in *Caring for People* (DoH, 1989a). No one was required to assess whether a person really needed residential or nursing home care. We have noted that this issue was a cause of concern to the Audit Commission and featured in the Griffiths Report, and according to Lewis and Glennerster (1996, p. 8) it is crucial to understanding the subsequent reforms: 'They were driven by the need to stop the haemorrhage in the social security budget and to do so in a way which would minimise political outcry and not give additional resources to the local authorities themselves'. Lewis and Glennerster argue that, 'What was new in the 1980s was the runaway cost of giving families what amounted to an open cheque book to buy residential and nursing home care – the most expensive kinds of alternatives available. No government could have let such a situation continue' (ibid., p. 195). Their view is that the government's prime objective was to check public spending and if possible reduce it. For those with the resources to pay then they would have to continue to pay the care home fees until their resources were substantially reduced.

The development of a mixed economy of care

A second policy goal of the Conservative government was to develop a market in social care. How this might be done was left largely to the local social service authorities. They were provided with a 'special transitional grant' to cover the costs of implementing the community care changes. Social service authorities were expected to establish a purchaser/provider split and 85 per cent of the special transitional grant money had to be directed towards independent providers. This had a considerable impact on the development of independent social care provision (Wistow *et al.*, 1996; Lewis and Glennerster, 1996) and the social care market. Lewis and Glennerster go so far as to write that 'The most significant central government intervention in the field of community care was the imposition of the 85 per cent rule late in 1992' (ibid., p. 200). A further boost to the social care market was provided by a Department of Health directive (LAC(92)27), which gave individual users the right to enter the home of their choice, within certain financial limits. A later directive (LAC(93)4) required the social service authorities to consult the independent sector when preparing community care plans. There thus developed a market in social care, accompanied by growing acceptance of the idea (Wistow *et al.*, 1996). Different organisational structures evolved but all adapted to the purchaser/provider split, the increased amount of independent provision and the regulation of this provision through contracts. More detail on the development of the mixed economy of care is given in Chapter 3.

Achieving a seamless service

The dual objectives of controlling expenditure and creating a 'market' of care were the main objectives but there were also others, such as the development of a seamless service, care management, and the development of quality assurance systems. Throughout the postwar period, problems arose in respect of different agencies working together well and effectively, and joint working from the mid 1970s only led to some marginal improvements in some areas. The problem was often exacerbated by the existence of different geographical boundaries for the healthcare and social care authorities.

The 1990 *Policy Guidance* (DoH, 1990) referred to the aim of 'seamless care', suggesting that users should not be conscious of organisational divisions in the delivery of services. Adding to the previous problems were the problems thrown up by the purchaser/provider split within social service authorities. Perhaps more typical than a 'seamless service' was a pattern of buck-passing and cost-shunting between agencies, with consequent frustrations for service users. Government policy since 1997 has put even more emphasis on achieving a seamless service and to this end a number of incentives have been introduced, as well as some legislative changes. Chapter 5 deals with this in more detail.

Care management

Care management was introduced as a policy objective and local authorities had to have it in place by 1993. This involved arranging packages of community services that would enable people to remain at home rather than go into residential care. Care management was a new way of working and was intended to provide an effective service to those in greatest need. It had been suggested in the Griffiths Report and was seen as an important part of the changes in *Caring for People* (DoH, 1989a). The form taken by assessment and care management was secondary to the government's main purpose and this partly explains why there has been considerable variation in the way in which it has developed. Care packages, usually commissioned by social workers or care managers from 'agencies' who provide the service, is now a common and familiar part of the community care territory. Chapter 4 looks at care management in detail.

Quality assurance

A fifth policy objective was to set up a system of quality assurance. By April 1991, each social service authority had to have a complaints procedure and an inspection unit to inspect all homes for adults. This was the first step towards ensuring that all authorities had some basic mechanisms for checking on quality and rectifying problems. Into the new century, local authorities lost their inspectorial function. Each part of the United Kingdom set up an independent inspectorate or commission to check on quality and standards. Both health and social services staff have had to contend with large amounts of guidance, targets, performance indicators, and varied quality assurance systems. Commenting on Labour's 1998 White Paper, Parton wrote,

> 'It is primarily concerned with regulating local authority departments through a series of supervisory and monitoring bodies, with setting new standards and targets with which to measure performance, and for agencies to enforce these, and with establishing a new system for placing social care workers under the guidance of new regulatory bodies'. (Parton, 2004, p. 36)

How did local authorities respond to the funding pressures?

It was argued above that curbing social security spending was at the heart of the government's policy. The community care measures imposed on the local authorities were used as a way of limiting or capping the increasing social security spending. However, within a matter of months, many local authorities were finding it hard to meet the financial demands of community care. They responded to the funding problem in a number of ways, including lobbying the government, expecting more from the voluntary sector and ensuring that service users were receiving their full benefit entitlement. The main mechanisms they used to stay within their budgets are outlined below.

The tightening of eligibility criteria

Local authorities were asked to set up eligibility criteria so that staff and users could be clear about who was entitled to a service. A typical set of criteria is shown in Box 1.4.

Box 1.4   An example of eligibility criteria

- Category 1, high priority: an emergency or crisis point has been reached.
- Category 2, medium priority: a high level of need is assessed.
- Category 3, low priority: a need appears to exist and a response from the social service authority is appropriate.
- Category 4, non-priority: help may be desirable but it is not essential that it comes from the social service authority.

One way of coping with budgetary pressure was to tighten the way the eligibility criteria were operated. For example, in year 1 (1993–94) an authority may have had sufficient resources to respond to categories 1, 2 and 3. However, in later years it may have only been able to respond to categories 1 and 2. If financial pressures continued to mount, it would have to look again at the criteria – one strategy is obviously to restrict its response to situations in category 1. At the end of 1994 Gloucestershire County Council announced that it could provide emergency care only to people who were 'at immediate physical risk' – presumably category 1 of their eligibility criteria.

The Audit Commission urged local authorities to set eligibility criteria to fit their budget allocations. Eligibility criteria 'should be set at such a level that authorities can meet the needs of those who qualify and still keep within budget' (Audit Commission, 1996, p. 10). It is through the eligibility criteria that resources are rationed, that is, 'need' is equated with 'resources available'. This mechanism severely limited the idea that provision could be determined either by need or by the right to services.

Many social service authorities also made use of decision-making 'panels'. By channelling all requests through such panels, a tight check could and can be maintained on resources. Many practitioners now spend a lot of time 'managing rationing' rather than providing direct care.

The Labour government acknowledged this problem in *Modernising Social Services*: 'Eligibility criteria are getting ever tighter and are excluding more and more people who would benefit from help but who do not come into the most dependent categories' (DoH, 1998a, para. 2.3). This raised the question of whether there could be an alternative to the situation of tighter and tighter eligibility criteria providing services to the few (the targeted). There has been a move towards a more standardised system of eligibility criteria and this is looked at in Chapter 4. However, the principle of using eligibility criteria as a means of saving money, balancing budgets and targeting those in greatest need remains central (DoH, 2002d).

Cut current services

Some authorities responded to their funding problems by cutting services. A key aim of the reforms was to focus provision on those defined as in the greatest need. This necessarily meant that people with less acute needs have had the services they receive reduced. For example, up to 1,500 people were affected in September 1994 when Gloucestershire Social Services cut its community care services to reduce its overspend. The necessity of Gloucestershire cutting its social services budget by £2.5 million and its inability to raise extra resources were due to the rate capping procedures of the time. The issue at stake was whether local councils should take their resources into account or whether they had a 'duty to care'. This tension between needs and resources is well-illustrated by the Gloucestershire judgment, described in Box 1.5.

Box 1.5 The Gloucestershire judgment

One of the 1,500 affected by the social service cuts in Gloucestershire in 1994 was 78-year-old Michael Barry, who lived alone at home, could walk only with a zimmer frame due to a fractured hip, had suffered a stroke, several heart attacks and some sight loss, and had no contact with his family. Gloucester Social Services withdrew all help with cleaning and laundry, although they continued to provide help with shopping and meals on wheels.

Michael Barry and a number of others applied for judicial review of the decision. The case went to the High Court, the Appeal Court and eventually the House of Lords. In March 1997, the Law Lords ruled by a majority of three to two that Gloucestershire County Council was within the law in withdrawing home help services from this elderly disabled man. The majority of judges backed the council's argument that resources, as well as need, should be taken into account when deciding on the provision of services.

Lord Nicholls wrote of the need to 'recognise that needs for services cannot sensibly be assessed without having some regard to the cost of providing them. A person's need for a particular type or level of services cannot be decided in a vacuum from which all considerations of cost have been expelled' (transcript of judgment).

The dissenting voices were those of Lord Lloyd and Lord Steyn. Lord Lloyd said that Gloucestershire had been placed in an 'impossible position' by government spending cuts. 'The solution lies with the Government. The passing of the Chronically Sick and Disabled Persons Act 1970 was a noble aspiration. Having willed the end, Parliament must provide the means' (transcript of judgment).

Limiting the cost of care packages

Most authorities put a limit on the care packages they are prepared to fund, although there is variation between authorities. In a study in England and Wales, Wright (2000) found that 69 per cent of social services departments set a fixed ceiling on how much they would spend on any one person. Once it becomes more expensive for the authority to fund someone living in the community than it would be to contribute to their residential or nursing care, then this may indicate the top end of any package that is likely to be funded for an extended period. Someone in a residential or nursing home pays towards the cost through his or her pension or income support and receives a small allowance for personal expenditure. Thus, the net cost to a local authority of providing a place in an average-cost residential home after the resident's own payments are taken into account will be somewhat less that the actual fees of the home. It is this sort of figure that many authorities set as the maximum they would pay for a package of care within the community. If money was very short, this limit might be reduced further. As an alternative, some authorities have limited the number of home care hours they would provide for any one person. The outcome of either method would usually hasten entry to a care home.

Modernising Social Services acknowledged the problem: 'The evidence is that many authorities are setting a financial ceiling on their domiciliary care packages, particularly in services for older people, which can lead to premature admissions to care homes when care at home would have been more suitable' (DoH, 1998a, para. 2.7).

Where care packages involve placement in a residential or nursing home, a further way of responding to funding pressures has been to cut the amount paid to the independent providers. One consequence of this is that the latter may feel forced to cut back on activities and other provisions for residents. Many homes have complained that the money received has not been enough and several have argued that they have gone out of business because of it.

Reviewing charging policy

Section 17 of the Health and Social Services and Social Security Adjudication Act 1983 gave local authorities the power to recover 'such charge (if any) as they consider reasonable'. The power to charge is discretionary but in a survey the charity Mencap found that 95 per cent of local authorities in England and Wales were charging for non-residential community care services (Mencap, 1999). Charges were introduced or increased for a range of service provisions during the 1990s as a means of raising further money. Mencap argued that many families were in the Catch-22 position of not being able to cope without services but being unable to afford them. Charging policies and charging levels varied considerably between authorities. *Modernising Social Services* deemed this as unacceptable (DoH, 1998a, para. 2.29) and steps were taken to establish greater equity between local authorities. Research by Age Concern England (Thompson and Matthews, 2004) indicated more consistency and fairness for those on low income but little evidence of fairness for those on middle incomes or those with some capital.

A range of people, groups and organisations are involved in community care, including family carers, neighbours, local organisations, housing authorities, voluntary organisations and private organisations. Coverage is given to these later in the book, especially in chapters 2 and 3. Special mention in this introductory chapter, however, needs to be given to the health services. While local authorities have faced considerable changes in relation to community care, big changes have also taken place in the health services and many of these have affected community care. This is the next focus of our discussion.

Healthcare changes

Social care is only one element of the range of services that make up the jigsaw puzzle of community care. The NHS&CC Act 1990 shook up both the National Health Service and social service authorities in dramatic ways, mapping out a different and rather uncertain future for them and introducing new concepts to both: purchaser/provider, contracts, markets, consumerism and user rights.

Most of the NHS&CC Act 1990 was actually concerned with changes to the health service. The background to these changes was contained in a government review of the health service and a White Paper, *Working for Patients* (DoH, 1989b). The government wanted an internal market to be introduced into the NHS, believing that this would encourage managers to be more efficient. In this internal market, each hospital or NHS community service unit would compete against others for contracts to care for a certain number of patients. In private industry such competition is supposed to keep prices low. The same principle was now applied to the health service and use of the term purchaser/provider split became commonplace.

Hospitals and NHS community services were encouraged to become independent trusts within the NHS, which gave them a good deal of freedom to organise their own affairs. Community nurses were increasingly employed by community trusts. Market ideas were also extended to GPs, who could opt to become budget-holding GPs, able to control their own budgets and negotiate with hospitals for the best deal for their patients. Practice nurses were increasingly employed in GP surgeries under these new fund-holding arrangements. In this way, the 'new' NHS evolved through the creation of more trusts and GP fundholders.

During the early 1990s, the NHS continued to withdraw from long-term care for older people. Once patients were no longer seen by the medical profession as in need of medical care, any subsequent care was seen as 'social care', organised and paid for by social service authorities or the individuals themselves, subject to means-testing. Long-stay hospital accommodation for older people continued to be phased out. The early 1990s saw the growth of considerable tension between social service authorities and health services over who was responsible for what (this is looked at in Chapter 3). In 1995, some clarification was provided in a government circular (LAC(95)5), which stated that the NHS had responsibilities for continuing care in the areas of rehabilitation and recovery, palliative health-care, respite care and community health service support. However, this has remained a troublesome issue lacking clarity as we shall see in Chapter 3.

The Labour government's approach to health was outlined in the White Paper, *The New NHS: Modern, Dependable* (DoH, 1997a). In broad terms, the internal market was to be done away with and the NHS would work in a more collaborative way towards more 'integrated' care. Similar proposals were put forward in separate White Papers for Scotland, Wales and Northern Ireland. Since then there have been numerous policy documents and changes that have tried to move forward a 'modernisation' agenda. A key element of this agenda has been the setting of targets and the need to meet them. In England, the *NHS Plan* of 2000 (DoH, 2000b) set a framework for ten years. Much more money was put into the NHS and this impacted by, for example, reducing waiting lists, improving services for people with heart disease and cancer and recruiting more staff. Encouragement was given to the private sector to provide more services within the NHS and 'patient choice' became a key theme of policy. Two parts of the government's health strategy with particular relevance for community care will be picked out – primary care and preventive healthcare.

Continuing emphasis on and development of primary care

The terms primary, secondary, continuing and intermediate care are sometimes used as a shorthand description of health service provision. Secondary care is broadly taken to mean hospital provision and historically the vast majority of NHS money has gone into hospital care. Continuing care is care that may be needed after hospital medical treatment and includes respite care, rehabilitative care and palliative care. Intermediate care has been a relatively recent development and will be described at the end of this section. Primary care is community-based care and is the first stage of healthcare usually involving GPs, practice nurses, health visitors, district nurses and community therapists.

During the 1990s, it was increasingly stressed that primary care should be given priority in terms of health service provision. The Labour government elected in 1997 continued the emphasis on primary healthcare. Primary Care Groups were set up (in Wales these were called Local Health Groups and in Scotland Local Healthcare Cooperatives), GP fund-holding as such came to an end and the new organisations were led by GPs and community nurses. As a result, GPs had a central role in a further shift away from hospital care and towards healthcare in the community. This development moved forward rapidly with Primary Care Groups becoming Primary Care Trusts (PCTs) in England and Local Health Groups becoming Local Health Boards in Wales. In Scotland, Community Health Partnerships have a somewhat similar role and are the successor bodies to Local Healthcare Cooperatives.

Box 1.6   Community Health Partnerships

In Scotland, Community Health Partnerships have been set up as statutory bodies to manage in a collaborative way community-based health provision. Each partnership covers a population of between 100,000 and 150,000 people. In some areas, these partnerships have also taken on social care, moving towards linking together health and social care budgets. The Scottish government has given a big emphasis to joint working and collaborative working and given much less emphasis to the development of markets and private sector provision.

In England, the *NHS Plan* (DoH, 2000b) saw the projected PCTs as pivotal to the reform process. By 2002, these were established throughout England with enhanced funding and strong backing from the government. They quickly became the main health commissioning organisations for localities. The government also expanded the scope for closer cooperation between the health and social service authorities through, for example, the pooling of budgets. This is examined in more detail in Chapter 5.

One example of this closer cooperation and closer working at the local level is in the area of 'intermediate care' for older people. The *NHS Plan* (DoH, 2000b) set out a programme to promote independence for older people. Intermediate care was a key element of that programme and was central to the modernisation agenda. There has been a major investment of money in this area. Intermediate care is a range of integrated services that promote faster recovery from illness, prevent unnecessary acute hospital admission, support timely discharge and maximise independent living (DoH, 2001c). It is supposed to last at most for six weeks and often lasts for less time than this. In the past, aspects of this have often been referred to as 'rehabilitation services'. In Scotland, there has been a similar emphasis but the language of 'integrated care' is sometimes used (Petch, 2003).

An emphasis on preventive health

The Labour government of 1997 put particular emphasis on public health issues. It appointed a public health minister and the previous government's 'Health of the Nation' strategy was replaced by a new strategy called 'Our Healthier Nation'. The four countries of the United Kingdom each published a Green Paper on the way forward. These acknowledged the growing inequality between the health status of the rich and the poor, which the previous government had failed to do. This was a significant and important step forward. The new approach also stressed the importance of having a community work or community action element in its strategy. 'Our Healthier Nation' set targets for improved public health in relation to cancer, strokes, accidents and mental health, to be achieved by 2010. Part of the strategy was also devolved responsibility for tackling specific problems to the areas where they occurred. Three particular settings for action were identified as schools, workplaces and neighbourhoods. The English

White Paper, *Saving Lives: Our Healthier Nation* (DoH, 1999b), added details to the proposals and set a target of saving 300,000 lives by 2010. It stressed the important role to be played by nurses and health visitors in health promotion. A second English White Paper, *Choosing Health: Making Healthy Choices Easier* (DoH, 2004b), gave emphasis to tackling obesity, smoking, alcohol consumption and sexual health. There was a considerable emphasis on different organizations coming together to improve the situation. Progress was to be achieved by varied local partnerships – joining the NHS with local government, the voluntary and community sector and business communities.

Preventive measures have obvious implications for community care. The incapacitation of people through strokes and heart disease is a major factor in the demand for community care services, so the prevention of strokes, heart disease or accidents reduces the pressure on community care resources. A lower incidence of cancer reduces the need for palliative care. The human and social cost of mental distress is enormous and all attempts at prevention are important. Effective 'harm-reduction' policies in relation to drugs results in fewer cases of HIV/AIDS and hepatitis B and C.

These preventive initiatives are important not only in themselves but also in experimenting with new relationships at the local level between workers and between professional workers and their communities. There are lessons to be learnt for wider community care from the work in preventive health.

Caring for People (DoH, 1989a) included a commitment to 'promote positive and healthy lifestyles among all age-groups through health education and the development of effective health surveillance and screening programmes' (ibid., p. 11), but the overall aim of the community care changes was essentially to target those in greatest need. However, this emphasis is changing with increasingly there being a vision of an overarching, inclusive framework that provides better links between community care and preventive health (DoH, 2005b). The language of integrated care is increasingly used and Box 1.7 gives a sense of the way policies may develop over future years.

Box 1.7 *Which way forward?*

The English government published a Green Paper in 2005 (DoH, 2005b). Its title, *Independence, Well-being and Choice*, summed up the key themes of the way the government saw the way forward. Choice and independence were indeed central to future thinking. Plans were set out for service users to be able to choose and buy the care they need. Outcomes were outlined which can be summarised as:

- more choice and control for service users
- improved quality of life, including health and economic well-being
- protection of personal dignity and freedom from discrimination and harassment

Proposals are set out to increase the use of self assessment, direct payments and individual budgets. There was to be greater emphasis on preventive services and greater use of strategic commissioning. New approaches to care management were suggested with care brokers, or facilitators or navigators. These ideas were incorporated into a joint health and social care White Paper published early in 2006. Called *Our Health, Our Care, Our Say: A New Direction for Community Services* (DoH, 2006), it set out to achieve four goals in its vision:

- Provide better prevention services with earlier intervention
- Enable people to have more choice and a louder voice
- Tackle inequalities to improve access to community services
- Provide more support for people with long term conditions

The White Paper acknowledged that health and social care services work together and aimed to build on this for the future with a programme that consolidated joint working and moved towards more integrated care.

The wider context

When discussing community care it is possible to keep a narrow focus on legislative requirements and practitioner issues to do with care management and coping with limited resources. Community care can be interpreted as being limited to targeting those in greatest need of care packages. The changes within social service authorities (usually a split between child care and adult care), the emphasis on the market economy and the purchaser/provider split, and the focus on individuals has meant that the provision of community care has had a tendency to be reduced to the provision of individual assessments of packages and has lost touch with the wider processes. There is a need to see community care in the wider context of societal and social policy influences.

Traditionally, healthcare has also often been very much located in individual diagnosis and treatment, although public health approaches have usually taken a much wider perspective. In the nineteenth century, charitable welfare organisations were concerned with identifying and helping the 'deserving' poor, and there seem to be parallels between this and the community care guidance on 'targeting those in greatest need'. Just as in the nineteenth century there were those who argued against the philosophy of individualistic help to the deserving poor, there is a need in the present era to reject a definition of community care that is solely about those in greatest need. Now, as then, there are wider issues that need to be addressed.

Social care and healthcare always takes place in the broader political context. With the individualising process inherent in the community care changes, it has sometimes been easy to lose sight of this. Mills argued more than forty years ago that the sociological imagination was important in making connections between 'personal troubles' and 'the public issues of social structure' (Mills, 1959). The need for the sociological imagination to make these links is as important in the new millennium as it was for Mills in the 1950s.

Practitioners need to understand these 'public' issues and try to incorporate this understanding into their practice, difficult though this can sometimes be. These issues include the growth of poverty; race discrimination; the exclusion of mental health service users; domestic violence; discrimination against and homophobia towards gay and lesbian people; the exclusion and stigmatisation of people with learning difficulties; and discrimination against older people. There is a desire among many practitioners to design a practice method that addresses these issues rather than ignores them.

For example, race discrimination was not addressed in the Audit Commission's report of 1986 and was only briefly addressed in the Griffiths Report (1988) and the White Paper (DoH, 1989a). The NHS&CC Act 1990 was silent on race, despite many issues of concern (Ahmad and Atkin, 1996). A report on eight authorities by the Social Services Inspectorate in 1998, *They Look After Their Own, Don't They?* (DoH, 1998b), indicated that although some progress had been made, black and ethnic minority older people were subject to significant disadvantage in gaining access to community care services. Box 1.8 indicates that it is acknowledged up to government level that much needs to be changed within, for example, the mental health services.

Box 1.8   David Bennett

In 1998, Mr David Bennett died in a medium secure psychiatric ward in Norwich. He was a 38-year-old African-Caribbean who had been diagnosed with schizophrenia. On the evening of his death, he had been racially abused by another patient. An inquiry into his death, under Sir John Blofeld, a retired high court judge, found in 2004 that Bennett was held face down on the floor for 25 minutes by at least four mental health nurses.

The Blofeld report said that the Department of Health gave a poor standard of treatment to patients from ethnic minorities (Norfolk, Suffolk and Cambridgeshire Strategic Health Authority, 2003). Twenty-two recommendations were made and the inquiry called for the government to accept that the services were affected by 'institutional racism'.

A report by the National Institute for Mental Health (2003) had outlined the evidence in relation to services and outcomes for black and ethnic communities in England and had outlined ideas for change. The government drew on this report and the Blofeld Report in drawing up an action plan for reform both inside and outside services (DoH, 2005a). The government committed itself to a five-year plan to halt racial discrimination in the NHS mental health services in England.

Box 1.8 indicates acknowledgement within government of racism and discrimination within the mental health services. This is just chosen as one area of which practitioners need to be aware. Similarly, for example, practitioners need to have the imagination to confront the homophobia faced by gay or lesbian service users within the context of a society that has historically discriminated against them and made few attempts to ensure that services and organisations are sensitive to their needs (Brown, 1998).

There are very varying views on the merits of the community care changes of the early 1990s. However, they did give attention to some neglected groups of people and this was welcomed. In the late 1990s, the Labour government put the tackling of 'social exclusion' at the centre of its programme. Many community care service users experience social exclusion and this emphasis provided the opportunity to bring both services and users more into the mainstream. 'Social exclusion' is now a commonly used term to describe social division in European societies. It has been used a good deal in relation to the social policy of the European Union. In this broad area health and social care practitioners can play a part through ideas/practice on empowerment and community work. Community work approaches have much to offer to tackle exclusion and bring about social inclusion.

There is renewed interest in the regeneration of the poorest areas, which often have a high proportion of community care concerns. For example, there are high concentrations of people with mental health problems or drug/alcohol problems in poor areas of cities. Problems that afflict whole communities are not best addressed by individualistic actions by reactive services (Barr et al., 1997, 2001). While there has been a history of regeneration policies going back forty years, during the 1980s and the early 1990s the emphasis was on economic objectives and the role of the private sector, with the aim of increasing inward investment into certain areas in need of regeneration.

More recent policies and approaches have included a social dimension with a strong emphasis on the need for a set of policies to tackle social exclusion. Government policy documents have stressed the strong association between ill health and low income (DoH, 1999b). The attention given by the government to poverty, exclusion and poor neighbourhoods has opened up opportunities for practitioners to relate their practice to these wider issues. These developments represent some recognition of the 'structural' issues that affect community care. However, the problems are deep-rooted and Wilkinson (2005), for example, has amassed a large amount of information from all over the world to show the impact on health of inequality.

Practice issues

This chapter has given something of an overview and indicated further coverage in later chapters. It has outlined the very considerable changes in the health and social care services, and practitioners have had to find a new role for themselves within the remit of these changes. Despite some of the frustrations caused by the changes, they have focused welcome attention on groups that have been traditionally neglected. The new structures do enable more people to remain in their own home in the community and this is what the vast majority want to do.

The changes have certainly raised some fundamental questions about the role of practitioners. Within local authorities, social workers (often called care managers) have seen a big change in their role. Since my own return to practice, I have found much more emphasis on people remaining in the community and there are more resources to enable this to happen. Services may vary in quality but there is greater variety and flexibility. Some interesting and innovative initiatives exist. Equally, some practitioners would complain about the large amount of paperwork; the domination of their day and practice by the needs of computer systems and by performance indicators; the difficulty of practising social work skills; and the frustration of working within the eligibility criteria. It has been difficult to find a path through the paperwork, the demands of technology, the increased bureaucracy and personal stress. A number of writers have tried to make connections between these changes and the 'wider' societal changes and context covered in the previous section (for example, Parton and O'Byrne, 2000).

Community nursing and workloads also changed dramatically during the 1990s (Audit Commission, 1999). Community nurses are managing complicated treatments in the community that previously took place in hospitals, and they are nursing far more terminally ill people at home.

Most of the bathing and putting-to-bed provision is now done by home care services (ibid.)

This chapter has suggested that there are links to be made by practitioners between personal troubles and public issues (Mills, 1959), hard though it can be to raise one's focus above the pressing individual needs that present themselves. This links into the possibilities of anti-discriminatory practice and the debates on it (Thompson, 2006). There is also a developing literature on what a 'critical social work' practice would look like in what is sometimes described as a post-modern period (e.g., Pease and Fook, 1999; Fook, 2002; Davies and Leonard, 2004).

Since the election in 1997 of the Labour government, health and social care agencies have had to adapt to a large number of changes and initiatives. As the new government's policies took shape, certain themes emerged, such as interagency working, preventive health, the tackling of exclusion and user involvement. These topics are covered in chapters 5 and 7. Links should be made by practitioners between the users of community care services and some of these policies, especially with regard to social exclusion, regeneration and preventive health.

What is needed is imaginative practice that works with and alongside the community and uses limited resources (such as practitioners' time and energy) to good effect. It is hoped that this book will play a small part in providing ideas and encouragement.

Further reading

Community care practice has a background in legislation, guidance and the decisions of the law courts. Two guides to this are:

Clements, L. (2004) *Community Care and the Law*, 3rd edn (London: Legal Action Group). A good, comprehensive guide to the law in this area. This gives coverage of England and Wales.

Mandelstam, M. (2005) *Community Care Practice and the Law*, 3rd edn (London: Jessica Kingsley). Written in relation to England but each chapter contains pointers to the provision in the rest of the United Kingdom.

Means, R., S. Richards and R. Smith (2003) *Community Care: Policy and Practice*, 3rd edn (London: Palgrave). This is a useful overview and background study of community care.

World Wide Web sites

The Department of Health site provides a lot of information. In particular, circulars and the full text of recent Green Papers and White Papers can be studied at www.dh.gov.uk

Policy changes in Scotland can be found at www.scotland.gov.uk in Wales at www.cymru.gov.uk and in Northern Ireland at www.nio.gov.uk

The Social Care Institute for Excellence (SCIE) was launched in 2001 under the Care Standards Act 2000 as part of the government's drive to improve social care and therefore as part of its 'modernisation' programme. Its web site is a source of much information about aspects of social care and good practice in social care: www.scie.org.uk

SCIE is home for a database of much information on community care at www.scie-socialcareonline.org.uk

CHAPTER 2

Care Within the Community

Chapter summary

This chapter covers:

- The interweaving of formal and informal care.
- The different ways in which service agencies respond to carers and care receivers.
- Data on carers from surveys and research studies.
- An analysis of why people care and an exploration of the complexity of caring.
- The tension between a focus on carers and a focus on independent living.
- The possible 'commodification' of care.
- Carers and assessment.

Introduction

It was stressed in Chapter 1 that the vast majority of community care has been and is provided by informal carers. This chapter focuses on the role of carers. The provision of care within the community is a fascinating topic and all readers will have some information and insights from their own lives upon which to draw. Many will be involved in caring or being cared for and can reflect on why it is done, how much is done, their feelings about it and their feelings about others doing less or more. Those without direct experience may have relatives or friends who can provide insights. The NHS&CC Act 1990 itself largely ignored carers but the policy guidance *Community Care in the Next Decade and Beyond* (DoH, 1990) provided some guidance about taking the preferences of carers into account and indicated that in some circumstances there might be a need for carers to receive a separate assessment. Pressure for better legislation resulted in The Carers (Recognition and Services) Act 1995, which came into force in April

1996 throughout the United Kingdom. This was primarily concerned with informal carers who provided or intended to provide regular and substantial care to others. It was left to local authorities themselves to define 'regular' and 'substantial', although 20 hours each week was often taken as an indication of substantial care (Heron, 1998). Practitioners have had to struggle with what these terms mean because it is not just time spent caring that has an impact. Having a job or having other family responsibilities may be part of the picture (DoH, 2005c, para. 22). Carers who meet the local authority's criteria have a right to an assessment of their ability to care and to continue caring. The results of the assessment must be taken into account when making decisions about services for the service user. Importantly, the Act recognised the contribution and particular circumstances of young carers.

In 1999, the Labour government published a national strategy for carers in England called *Caring About Carers* (DoH, 1999a), which acknowledged the contribution made by carers and outlined ways in which more support and help could be given to them. The Scottish government published its own strategy (Scottish Executive, 1999a) and the Welsh strategy was published shortly afterwards (National Assembly for Wales, 2000b). The Carers and Disabled Children Act 2000 applied only in England and Wales. This gave carers a right to receive an assessment when they requested it even if the service user had refused an assessment or services. It also made possible direct payments for carers, a voucher scheme for carers (issued to enable them to have a break from caring) and more services for carers. The Carers (Equal Opportunities) Act 2004 also applied only to England and Wales and placed a duty on local authorities and health authorities to inform carers of the right to an assessment in their own right (this duty had already been introduced in Scotland and Northern Ireland). When undertaking an assessment, councils need to consider the carer's wish to work, undertake education, training or leisure activities. The Act also made law the duty of cooperation between local health, education and housing authorities in the planning and provision of services for carers.

As suggested in Chapter 1, it is again recommended that readers turn to web sites for recent developments and for details specific to the country that they are living in or working in. The web sites relevant to the four countries were given at the end of Chapter 1 and these have within them information on legislation, policy and guidance on carers. Another option is to look at the four web sites relating to Carers UK that are given at the end of this chapter.

Carers UK (formerly the Carers National Association) is the UK's leading organisation of carers. It provides information to carers and it puts carers in contact with a network of branches and groups throughout the United

Kingdom. It has played a significant role in raising awareness of carers' issues and in effectively lobbying government for change. This is a good example (of which there are many in community care) of collective issues of concern being addressed by small local organisations or a national voluntary organisation. The individual concerns of carers can be shared with others and channelled at the national level. Practitioners need to see beyond the individual and pay attention to these wider collectivities perhaps by assisting the development of a group or helping a carer to join a group. Working with groups and collectivities in this way not only utilises the skills of community workers but also allows practitioners to make links between personal troubles and public issues (as advocated at the end of Chapter 1).

Hadley and Clough (1996, p. 207) argue that at the core of the Thatcherite project during the 1980s was the notion of 'the self-interested individual pursuing his or her own maximum good'. There are alternatives to this view, one being the idea of 'mutuality', as outlined by Holman (1993). Indeed it can be argued that the very basis of community care is such mutuality. Most care in the community is provided by informal carers, especially partners and adult children. Among the many reasons why people become involved are love, duty and obligation – the basic ingredients of mutuality. One example of this is given in Box 2.1.

Box 2.1   *Iris – Iris Murdoch and Alzheimer's disease*

Many books and films touch on aspects of community care and give us insights that we can learn from. The novelist Iris Murdoch developed Alzheimer's disease. Her husband John Bayley wrote about this experience (Bayley, 1998) and the story was turned into the beautifully acted film entitled *Iris*. The film covers Iris Murdoch's early life but its chief focus is on the five years between the diagnosis of the disease and her death. It gives a portrayal of the development of the disease on a creative and intelligent woman. It also shows the pressures on John Bayley, the main carer, as he tries to cope with the whole process — caring for her, nursing her and loving her. It shows a combination of love, duty and obligation.

A sensible system of community care needs to be based on this mutuality – to work with it and foster it. There has to be an interlinking of formal and informal care. Ideally this would be a balanced partnership without one exploiting the other. This can perhaps be obtained through the notion of 'interweaving' (Bulmer, 1987), where the formal services and the informal sector cooperate in a spirit of partnership and mutual trust, as described by Bayley in the early 1970s:

> 'The social services seek to interweave their help so as to use and strengthen the help already given, make good the limitations and meet the needs. It is not a question of the social services plugging the gaps but rather of their working with society to enable society to close the gaps.' (Bayley, 1973, p. 343)

The more recent language used here is the language of 'partnership' and a full view of partnership would involve the care receiver(s), the informal care giver(s) and the service provider(s).

The response of service agencies to carers

Partnership can have different meanings. The relationship between service provision, care receivers and carers is uncertain and ill defined. Twigg and Atkin (1994) draw on Twigg's (1989) earlier work and propose four models that help to disentangle this:

Carers as resources. In this model, agencies regard carers as a type of resource. Agencies focus mainly on dependent people or the cared for and informal carers are only a background to these. They are a vital resource but not the primary subject of the agency's concern. Thus concern for carer welfare in this model is very limited.

Carers as co-workers. In this model, agencies see themselves as working along-side and in parallel with carers. The main image here is one of 'interweaving', which was referred to above as an appropriate aim for practitioners. The model encompasses the carer's interests and well-being.

Carers as co-clients. Here the carer is seen as a client, as someone in need of help in his or her own right. This model tends to be applied to cases where a lot of care is needed and the carer is very stressed. The aim of intervention is to relieve carer strain, and the conflicts of interest between carer and care receiver are fully recognised.

The superseded carer. With the superseded carer the aim is not to support the care-giving relationship but to transcend or supersede it. There are two routes to this. One route starts with the disabled person and a desire to maximise his or her independence. The more this is achieved, the more the carer and the disabled person are freed from the caring relationship. The other route starts with concern for the carer and freeing him or her from the caring role.

In their overview of how health and social services staff respond to family carers, Twigg and Atkin (1994) suggest that there may be a tendency for medical staff to regard carers as a resource whereas social care professionals tend to be more aware of carers as co-clients. Consider the above models in relation to the case study in Box 2.2. What are the key issues in this case study? Do the models help to clarify the issues or suggest different approaches?

Box 2.2   Case study

Jim, an autistic young man in his twenties, has been looked after at home by his parents all his life. His parents have done most things for him. He is not able to cook for himself or shop and has very few relationships. Most of his time is spent watching television. Since leaving school there have been attempts to persuade him to attend a day centre but he usually refuses to go. Jim now says that he wants to leave home. His parents fear that he will not cope and will become isolated and depressed without their ongoing support.

Jim's scenario is very briefly sketched out and therefore only initial ideas can be drawn out. With the first model (carers as resources) the practitioner would focus on Jim, with the parents in the background as a resource depending on what was identified as being needed by and for him. In the second model (carers as co-workers) an alliance is likely between the carers and the practitioner, with Jim's expressed wishes being a little less to the fore than in the first model. With the third model (carers as co-clients) equal attention will be given to Jim and his parents. Assuming he wants help to live independently, then help will also be given to the parents in terms of helping them to adjust to the idea and its actuality. The fourth model (the superseded carer) seems rather similar but the idea is that eventually the care-giving relationship will become redundant. Jim will receive a lot of help to live independently, and a lot of support, counselling and assistance will be given to his parents to help them see their role differently. The models are simply a possible aid to analysis. Change may of course be very difficult as Jim and his parents may have quite set patterns of behaviour and views.

Factors that affect caring

All caring situations are influenced by the nature of social policies and practices as well as family and personal factors. This will be illustrated in this section by discussing demographic changes, changes in employment patterns and changes in marriage/living patterns.

The composition of the UK population in terms of age is changing quite dramatically. The two main reasons for this are the fall in the birth rate and the fact that people are living longer. It is expected that the number of people aged 65 and over in the United Kingdom will rise from 9.3 million in 2000 to 16.8 million by 2051. Those over 85 are expected to grow even faster from 1.1 million in 2000 to 4 million in 2051 – an increase of 255 per cent (Wittenberg *et al.*, 2004). While the fact that more people are living longer is to be welcomed, the figures do have implications for community care and for health and social services provision. These figures suggest that the rise in demand for family care and health/social services provision could be substantial. It is not clear how informal and formal systems of care will respond to these demographic pressures. There will be an increasing need for services for older people and for additional resources to fund them. In comparison with earlier generations, people nowadays have fewer children and grandchildren, hence the care of older people will be provided by a much smaller number of younger people than in the past.

A second factor affecting caring is the significant change in employment patterns. There has been a considerable increase in the number of married women participating in the labour market. Williams (2004a, p. 15) points out that between 1971 and 2001, the full-time employment rate of women with dependent children trebled and the part-time employment rate doubled. These trends have led to a rise in the number of 'dual worker' families in which both parents go out to work. It does seem likely that these employment factors will limit the number of adult daughters and sons who are prepared to take on significant caring roles (Finch, 1995, p. 61). A further factor in employment patterns is job mobility. Many people have to move in order to find a job, necessitating a choice between finding paid work or taking care of a dependent relative. These decisions are and will continue to be affected by how satisfactory caring alternatives are perceived to be.

A third factor affecting caring is the change in patterns of living. Some key points provided by Williams (2004a) are shown in Box 2.3.

Box 2.3   Changes in patterns of living

- Between 1971 and 2001 cohabitation trebled. In 2001 43 per cent of woman and 37 per cent of men aged 20–35 cohabited.
- About 40 per cent of children experience parental divorce by the time they are 16.

- Single parent households doubled between 1971 and 2001.
- About 40 per cent of births are outside marriage. There was an increase of this by five times in the 30 years before 2001.

The statistics in Box 2.3 indicate that family life in Britain is undergoing unprecedented change. Family care has been and still is the mainstay of community care. Although dramatic changes have occurred within the family, it is not necessarily the case that feelings of kinship and obligation will decline (Finch, 1995). However, it does seem likely that the pool of carers will decline and that there may be an impact on people's sense of duty and obligation, leading to less family care. This is not certain. Indeed, Williams (2004a) argues that although relationships are changing, levels of commitment have not diminished and people generally negotiate 'the proper thing to do'.

At the wider policy level, the Labour Party after 1997 gave considerable emphasis in its policies to the ethic of 'paid work'. Some (Williams, 2001, 2004a) have argued that this should be balanced by an ethic of 'care', involving a more public validation of the importance of care. Bunting has also argued that Labour gave great emphasis to welfare-to-work with an absence of the ethic of care. She argued that caring needed to be given more attention and prestige. 'More recognition is needed urgently for the care ethic that many millions (especially women) have built their lives around; an ethic that holds transformative, redemptive possibilities in relationships of dependence. From that would come a reappraisal of those who care, the value of their work – and better pay' (Bunting, 2004).

This section has looked at demographic changes, changes in employment patterns and changes in living patterns. These raise several issues and question in relation to the future of community care:

- Given the increase in the divorce rate, cohabitation and lone-parent families, what are the implications of this change when so much informal care is provided by spouses?
- Given the increase in births outside marriage, divorce and the number of stepchildren, what are the implications in terms of care by children? Will children provide as much informal care as in the past?
- With the changes in employment patterns and more women working, will women provide as much care as they have in the past?
- Will employers develop more flexible employment patterns to enable people to combine work and caring?
- With the demographically ageing population, will old people care or be able to care for very old people?

- With changing attitudes towards care, duty and obligation, to what extent will adults want to impose on or trouble their children?

Who are the carers?

There was a considerable growth of interest in and research on informal caring during the 1980s and the 1990s, providing us with some under-standing of the origins, incidence, patterns and experiences of carers (for example, Twigg, 1992; Allen and Perkins, 1995). During the early 1980s, there was a strong sense in the literature that community care was family care and that family care meant care by women (Finch and Groves, 1983). A number of studies of small samples seemed to confirm this picture (Lewis and Meredith, 1988; Ungerson, 1987).

The 1985 General Household Survey was the first large-scale study to include detailed information on Britain's carers. The results of the survey were published in 1988 in a report called *Informal Carers* (Green, 1988). The data, which were obtained from a nationally representative sample of 18,500 adults, indicated that there were about six million carers in Britain: 3.5 million women and 2.5 million men. The data generated a debate on 'who does the caring'. In particular, it raised the issue of men as carers because the percentage of male carers (12 per cent of men aged 16 and over were carers) was not a great deal lower than that for women as carers (15 per cent). This seemed to contradict much of the feminist writing on the issue. However, the statistics provided a simplified picture. In a re-analysis of the data it was shown that men were less likely to be the 'main' carer, were more likely to be devoting fewer than 20 hours a week to the task and were less likely to be involved in personal caring (Parker and Lawton, 1994).

These overall figures were confirmed by an analysis of 2,700 adult informal carers from the 1990–91 General Household Survey by Arber and Ginn (1995), who found that 10 per cent of men, compared with 13 per cent of women, were involved in some form of caring. Their analysis shows that:

- Men's caring contribution is substantial – especially in later life when men often care for their partner and unmarried men care for a parent within the same household.
- Men are less likely than women to provide care for someone in another household.
- Men carers undertake fewer hours of care each week.
- Men carers are less likely to be the main carer.

The data seemed to indicate that the question of caring and gender appeared to be less clear-cut than was often claimed during the 1980s. Gender is nevertheless an important variable and Dalley (1996, p. 13) has summarised this as 'Women tended to do more, more often and more intimately'.

In 1999, the government estimated that nine out of ten carers cared for a relative, with two out of ten caring for a partner or spouse and four out of ten caring for parents (DoH, 1999a). The 2001 Census indicated that there are six million carers throughout the United Kingdom, 10 per cent of the total population, or approximately 12 per cent of the adult population (Carers UK, 2005). Fifty-eight per cent of the carers were women and 42 per cent were men. The Census indicated that 1.25 million carers provided over 50 hours of care a week (ibid.). Carers UK has estimated that carers save Britain's economy £57 billion a year (Carers UK, 2002).

There are carers for all of the service user groups, including old people, disabled people, people who are dying, people with drug or alcohol abuse problems, people who have had a stroke, people with dementia, people with learning difficulties and people with mental health problems. While there are common features of caring in all these situations there are also distinctive aspects in terms of the particular reasons why caring is taking place. There is then considerable diversity among carers (Eley, 2003).

Since the mid-1990s, attention has been given to the presence and the needs of young carers. The 2001 census showed that there were 174,995 young people under the age of 18 in the United Kingdom who provide care, 13,029 of them providing care for 50 hours or more a week (Carers UK, 2005). The Carers (Recognition and Services) Act 1995 gave particular mention to young carers. They, along with adult carers, have to be assessed for their ability to provide or continue to provide care. The child care legislation and guidance in each country ensures that a range of services can be provided for children who are carers. There are now a number of projects around the United Kingdom devoted to meeting the needs of young carers, mostly run by the voluntary sector. Dearden and Becker (2004) conducted a survey of 6,178 young carers from 87 of these projects. Girls made up 56 per cent of the sample and 44 per cent were boys, with 56 per cent of young carers living in lone parent families. Two thirds of the young carers provided domestic help; 48 per cent provided general and nursing-type care; and 82 per cent provided emotional support. Eighteen per cent of young carers had been assessed (ibid.).

There is little published material on gay or lesbian carers, but because roughly 10 per cent of the population are gay or lesbian there is bound to be a proportion of gay and lesbian carers in the population who provide care for their partners. Manthorpe (2003) argues that caring within lesbian relationships has been neglected in social and healthcare studies and practice. Box 2.4 lists a number of the issues for workers and agencies that might arise from the need to provide services for gay and lesbian carers.

Box 2.4   *Developing services for gay and lesbian service users*

- In the light of discrimination and homophobia, how reluctant would the carers be to seek help? What steps could be taken to overcome this fear of discrimination and hostility?
- What should the publicity material of an agency say about its services to gay and lesbian carers?
- What would an equal opportunities policy look like in relation to gay and lesbian service users, and should special mention be made of gay and lesbian carers?
- In reality, how sensitive would the formal services be? What constitutes a sensitive service?
- Heterosexual workers may be discriminatory in attitude. What training would be appropriate for them?

The General Household Surveys have too small a sample of black and ethnic minority carers for any useful analysis. Chapter 1 mentioned the danger of the assumption that 'they look after their own' and that policy and service provision are equally appropriate for everyone. In an overview of the literature, Atkin and Rollings (1996, p. 78) argue that when caring responsibilities are taken on, the locus of care is usually the immediate family and the main responsibility falls on one family member, usually the woman. In this respect, they note that 'Asian and Afro-Caribbean families are no different from white families' (ibid.). Likewise they argue that 'the experience of care-giving among Asian and Afro-Caribbean carers is broadly similar to that of white people. The physical, emotional and financial consequences of caregiving affect all carers, irrespective of ethnic origin' (ibid., p. 85). The research study outlined in Box 2.5 illustrates this.

Box 2.5   *Do they look after their own? Informal support for South Asian carers*

The title above is the title of a research study that explored South Asian carers' experiences of informal support. It was a study of 105 male and female carers from the Punjabi Sikh, Gujarati Hindu, and Bangladeshi and Pakistani communities (Katbamna *et al.*, 2004). The authors list some of the factors that raise questions about an assumption that 'they look after their own':

- Strict immigration laws
- A growing preference for nuclear households
- Occupational mobility
- Housing problems
- The fragmentation of family networks for many

The authors argue that what has placed additional strains on support systems and family ties are:

- Social and economic pressures
- Changes in marriage and divorce practices
- Increase in the participation of women in the labour market

The analysis of carers' accounts suggested that the main carer had limited support both in nuclear and extended households. The authors argue that societal attitudes towards disability and the fear of obligation worked against seeking and accepting of help from wider social networks. It is concluded that the evidence does not support the assumption that there is a reserve of people who can be called on to provide support to carers in South Asian communities. The authors argue that their study reinforces the conclusions of other research, 'that South Asian carers as a group are no more likely than carers from other communities to be assured of support from wider kinship and social networks. In fact, the findings challenge the pervasive assumption and stereotype that South Asian people live in self-supporting extended families, and therefore, that the support of the social services is largely unnecessary' (ibid., p. 404).

Why people do the caring

Community care is a phrase that may conjure up images of a warm, concerned community. In reality, community care often means heavy pressures on one relative, often a female relative. This section explores why the relative does the caring and the motivations of love, duty and obligation.

There is no easy answer to why people engage in the care of others as there is a complex of motivating factors. Co-residency and marital relationship (whether male or female) are clearly important factors in determining the pattern of caring (Parker and Lawton, 1994; Qureshi and Walker, 1989; Finch and Mason, 1993). The issue of gender has been much explored in the literature. According to Dalley (1996), women are pushed into both 'caring about' and 'caring for' while it is acceptable for men just to 'care about'. Dalley argues that 'the whole of community care policies can be seen to be based on the supposition that women are naturally carers, while men are naturally providers' (ibid., p. 18). The altruism of women is presumed upon.

Approximately four out of five carers are family members (Green, 1988), and it is clear that family care underpins community care, regardless of ethnic background (Finch, 1989; Atkin and Rollings, 1993). This raises a range of interesting questions, such as how it is decided within families who should care, how much the caring is shared and the nature of the caring. People's sense of duty and obligation towards their relations helps to sustain them during the process of caring. At the same time their sense of obligation varies according to the situation and their circumstances. Whether the family will care, who within the family will care and how much care will be provided are all sensitive issues and need careful exploration. The message from research for practitioners is that factors such as altruism, obligation and duty make the issue of caring very complicated to untangle (Finch, 1989; Qureshi and Walker, 1989; Finch and Mason, 1993).

Finch, in her study *Family Obligation and Social Change* (1989), makes a number of interesting observations in this respect. She argues that help and support from relatives is based on duty and obligation: "The idea that kin support is founded, in whole or in part, upon duty and obligation, implies that there is 'something special' about social relationships which we have with kin, which makes them distinctively different from all other relationships" (ibid., p. 212).

If kin relationships are special, what is it that is distinctive about them? Finch looks at possible explanations and concludes that the distinctive feature of kin relationships is the question of morality, which puts relationships with kin on a different basis from those with other people (ibid., 1989, p. 236). She argues that four main principles determine who offers personal care (ibid., pp. 27–8):

- The marriage relationship is the most important and the spouse is a prime source of support.
- Second to the marriage relationship is the parent–child relationship.
- People who share the same household are often major sources of support. These often belong to the first two groups. This means that a child who continues to live at home is more likely to be seen as responsible for care than those who have moved away.
- Women are much more likely than men to provide personal care.

The following is the commonly assumed hierarchy of who should care, listed in order of importance (Qureshi and Walker, 1989, p. 126):

- Spouse
- Relative in lifelong joint household
- Daughter
- Daughter-in-law
- Son

- Other relative
- Non-relative

While the influence of duty and obligation is stressed, it is never simple. Finch (1989, ch. 5) argues that support within families cannot be understood just in terms of certain expectations of duty or obligation. When people give support and assistance to their relatives they are not simply acting in accordance with preordained rules, but are engaged in a process of actively working out what to do (ibid., p. 179). Some carers may have a clear idea of what they want to do and what they should do. For others there may be uncertainty, anxiety, hesitation and confusion. Practitioners should bear in mind the varied feelings that might be present. Good counselling skills may be appropriate to help them determine what they can do.

This idea of 'working things out' and 'negotiation' is developed further in *Negotiating Family Responsibilities* by Finch and Mason (1993). The authors argue that relatives do not engage in caring because of fixed rules of obligation or fixed ideas of duty, but rather as a result of complex processes of negotiation. What relatives do in terms of caring depends on relationships within families over time. A history of reciprocity and exchange is the most important factor in creating a sense of obligation. Thus, family history and biography interact, resulting in the development of commitment.

Finch and Mason argue that reciprocity is important, and central to their discussion of how reciprocity operates in practice is the concept of 'balance': 'Getting the balance right is a central part of negotiating responsibilities and commitments within kin groups' (ibid., p. 37). There are subtle processes of negotiation and adaptation between parties, and they strive to achieve a balance between offering help and having to ask for it.

The above are brief summaries of complex studies, but some lessons for practitioners can still be drawn:

- Be conscious of the likely hierarchy of obligations.
- Caring responsibilities will probably have been negotiated over time. Be sensitive to this and the history of their development.
- Caring relationships can often be delicate and fragile arrangements and it is important to tread carefully, but there may be times when counselling skills and facilitating family group meetings may be appropriate.

Finch and Mason (1993) note similarities between Asian and white respondents in respect of norms of social obligation. Ahmad (1996) notes the limited literature on family obligations in minority ethnic communities. He draws together some of the available literature and argues that there is a pattern of negotiation based on personal and moral identity, the history of the relationship, the closeness of ties, class, gender and place in the family hierarchy. He notes that there exists a common stereotype of the virtuous caring family, especially the Asian family, but argues that 'These stereotypes ignore both the diversity of perspectives and behaviour within an ethnic group and the similarities across ethnic groups' (ibid., p. 51). Ahmad stresses the need for more research in this area. He notes the system of obligation and reciprocity that is central to the migration process. In addition to the family itself, Ahmad refers to the *biraderi* (a wider kinship-based network in which reciprocal relationships are based on moral, financial and social obligation), which is an important source of identity and support (ibid., p. 55). Kin and *biraderi* networks have been important in both the immigration process and the settlement/employment process.

Caring is complex

The previous section looked at caring in terms of how kinship rules are negotiated. Nolan *et al.* (1996) stress that caring is a complicated activity and involves much more than practical tasks. People, for example, anticipate what may be needed or monitor vulnerable members of their family at a distance. These activities are elements of caring, although do not provide day-to-day support. This complexity needs to be recognised and acknowledged if good practice by practitioners is to emerge.

Nolan *et al.* (ibid.) suggest that interventions can be seen along a continuum ranging from facilitative to obstructive. The intention of the partnership is to facilitate the best outcome for both the carer and the cared-for. They write that the key determinant of successful facilitative intervention is that 'services are planned in conjunction with the carer and cared-for person to complement their needs. Such services are, unfortunately, not the norm' (ibid., p. 49).

There needs to be a partnership between carer and professional – they should complement each other and the professional may well have much to learn from the carer. Too often help is seen in practical and instrumental terms when there is a need for practitioners to be skilled at dealing with emotions such as loss, grief, anxiety, anger and resentment. These are some of the traditional human relationship skills of social work (often used by all community care workers) and there is an important role for them in community care.

Stress is often a central part of the carer's experience and different people have different abilities to cope with it. It is important for the assessor to try to understand the particular stressors affecting a carer. Nolan *et al.* point out that often the main criteria determining perceived stress by practitioners come from practical aspects of caring. They argue, however, that other factors are more important – such as the nature and quality of relationship, the range of behaviours from the cared-for person and the adequacy of financial resources. The message here for practitioners in respect of assessment is not simply to focus on the practical tasks of personal and domestic care but to include these other factors. Some ideas on this are contained in Box 2.6.

Box 2.6 Developing support for carers

Practitioners can help carers to cope by:

- identifying and reinforcing appropriate coping responses by the carer;
- identifying and seeking to reduce inappropriate coping responses;
- helping carers to develop new coping resources/responses;
- augmenting existing coping resources by building larger support networks.

Nolan et al. argue that services should substitute for carers only when the above interventions prove unsuccessful. They also argue that practitioners should adopt a more enabling role by working with carers as partners in ways that are sensitive to the carers' expertise (Nolan et al., 1996, p. 80).

While caring can be stressful, there is satisfaction to be gained from the caring role. The obvious point here for the practitioner is that minimising the stress and helping to maximise the satisfaction is important when thinking about intervention (ibid., p. 106).

The complexity of life history, of negotiated caring (Finch and Mason, 1993) and the varied stresses and satisfactions make any assessment time-consuming and require detailed attention to the family's history. Nolan et al. (1996) devote a chapter to the way in which caring can go through a series of stages. These stages they describe as building on the past; recognising the need; taking it on; working it through; reaching the end and a new beginning. A second book by the same authors elaborates further on this model (Nolan et al., 2003) by illustrating how the need for support varies over time. The authors stress how important it is to acknowledge and recognise this in order to offer the most appropriate help at the most appropriate time.

The tensions between a focus on carers and a focus on independent living

The main focus of this chapter so far has been on carers, but it is essential to consider the importance of cared-for persons being responsible for their own lives. Policies and practice that directly try to support, help and maintain family care may run counter to policies and practices that enable people to control their own lives and live independently. This issue was touched on in the case study in Box 2.2 and the subsequent discussion, where models 3 and 4 were applied to a young man trying to achieve independence. A theme stressed in writings on disability and dependence is the need for and ability of disabled people to control their own activities, environments and lives. This has perhaps been best articulated by Jenny Morris (1993) in relation to carers of disabled people.

Morris argues that by the end of the 1980s, the interests of the disability movement and the Carers National Association were in deep conflict with each other. She writes that 'The identification of informal carers as a social group with specific interests, accompanied as it has been by the social construction of the older and disabled people as "dependent", has tended to limit the opportunities for the interests of older and disabled people to be heard' (ibid., p. 37).

At the heart of her argument is the idea that policy and practice should not endorse dependence by focusing on the support of carers but rather should help disabled people to live independently in the community, through direct payments and money provided by the Independent Living Fund. The emphasis on carers may divert attention and resources away from this ideal. Morris decries the fact that the voice of the user is absent in the carers' movement and in much of the feminist writing on carers, which stresses the pressure on and oppression of carers. She argues that it is most important not to forget the civil and human rights of older people and disabled people. Likewise, Arber and Ginn (1991) argued that there is a great need for policies that recognise older people's rights as citizens and the contribution they have made and still make to society.

While support for carers is important, there is a strong case for arguing that the priorities of policy and practice need to be geared towards achieving and maintaining the independence of older and disabled people. This includes welfare benefits, for which hard choices might have to be made between increasing benefits to carers (such as the Carer's Allowance) or providing extra funds to disabled people to enable them to live independently. The argument is that dependence on carer support can be reduced by the purchase of personal assistants through the use of direct payments. This is an interesting area where policy and practice may at times conflict and choices have to be made. An appropriate balance is needed between the needs of carers and the achievement of rights for disabled people and older people. This subject is returned to in Chapter 7.

Is informal care becoming 'commodified'?

This chapter has argued that much care is and has been given by the informal sector. In the past it has been assumed that informal care is unpaid care. However this clear-cut boundary may be crumbling. Increasingly cash payments have become a part of informal care. Ungerson (2002) argues that the boundaries between unpaid care and paid care have been breaking down and this has happened through the increased use of cash payments. Anything that is delivered and paid for is defined as a commodity and so social care provision can increasingly be seen as a commodity that can be bought and sold. The increase in the payments for care Ungerson calls the 'commodification of care'.

Situations in the past that would have been left as unpaid informal care arrangements are having cash payments attached to them in one form or another. Drawing on policies and experiences from different counties, Ungerson (2002, p. 352) puts forward five types of situations where payments may be made for care. These are:

(1) Carer allowances that are paid for either through tax or social security systems.
(2) In some Scandinavian countries, 'proper' wages have been paid to carers. These are paid by the state or state agencies.
(3) Routed wages that are paid directly to care users who then pay their carers. In the United Kingdom, direct payments would be an example of this.
(4) Symbolic payments that are paid by care users to kin, neighbours and friends. For example, someone may receive an attendance allowance and make some payments or 'gifts' (informally and non-contractually) from it for care given.
(5) Volunteers who are paid an amount from voluntary organisations and local authorities to do some visiting.

There is a strong movement towards payment for care. Ungerson gives several reasons why this is happening. Carers, for example, have become organised and campaigned for more money for carers. Disabled people have campaigned for the development of direct payments schemes. 'New Right' arguments support this development through ideas of consumer choice and efficiency (lower cost). Increasingly it is clear therefore that cash is a part of what has traditionally been seen as the 'cash free' informal sector. People may now be paid for what they have done for free in the past. Another aspect of this blurring of boundaries is the way that paid workers can become to feel part of the employer's family. For example, Leece (2004, p. 217) found in her study examples of personal assistants doing unpaid jobs and working unpaid hours. A number of intriguing dimensions are added to the complex world of community care.

Carers and assessment

The Carers Act 1995 gave carers the right to assessment. The aim was to bring together the needs identified in two assessments (the Section 47 assessment of NH&SCC Act 1990 and the Carers Act 1995) into one care plan. The two key elements of the 1995 Act were the carer's right to ask for an assessment of their ability to care and the local authority's duty to take into account the results of this assessment when looking at what support to provide for the person cared for.

Under the 1995 legislation, carers who are engaged in substantial and regular caring have to be informed about their right to be assessed. These assessments may be conducted in the presence or absence of the service user. Carers should be told that, if they wish, their assessment can take place during a separate interview. Indeed, it is normally best to assume that this will be the case as there are a number of situations in which it would be preferable and sensible (Heron, 1998, p. 68). Conflicts of interests may emerge from the two assessments and the practitioner may be involved in negotiating around these differing positions.

Heron suggests a framework for a carer assessment. As with any assessment it is important to set carers at ease with some conversation or general open-ended questions, such as 'Could you tell me about the situation as you see it?' or 'Could you explain about any difficulties you are facing?' (ibid., p. 72). The assessors would then explore the carers' responsibilities in terms of what sort of tasks they perform, how often they are required to do them and how long they take. It is important to ascertain how much support is currently being provided, who provides it and how regular and frequent it is. There may also be other people who could help with the caring but are not currently doing so. An assessment would explore carers' other commitments and the impact of the caring on their lives. Once well settled into the interview, the issue should be broached of the carer's relationship with the person being cared for. Heron notes that 'In many cases this issue will be the crux of why they have requested a separate assessment' (ibid., p. 74). An exploration of the carer's expertise and strengths might be followed by an investigation of the support they are looking for and how they feel about caring and the future. The final stage of the assessment is designing a care plan for the user that takes account of the needs of the carer. Any care plan should detail the input by informal carers and a copy should be given to the user and the carer(s).

Each local authority has its own assessment form or procedures that have to be completed to trigger services. The topics within these provide a guide to any assessment process. However, government guidance has indicated that the process should be carer-centred and should not be a bureaucratic process based on ticking boxes. The assessment 'must focus on the outcomes the carer would want to see to help them in their caring role and maintain their health and well-being' (DoH, 2001a, p. 7).

Practitioners may tend to relate people's caring situations to situations of which they have had some personal experience. There is a danger here of over-identification, where practitioners assume that carers have similar feelings and emotions to ones they have had. However, practitioners may overlook some aspects of caring because they have not encountered them before, for example caring in a gay or lesbian relationship or where a young person is caring for an adult.

The Carers (Equal Opportunities) Act 2004 (England and Wales) ensures that all carers are made aware of their right to an assessment of their ability to provide care. The Act also expands on what needs to be considered by local authority's in an assessment – there is a duty requiring councils to consider the carer's wish to work, undertake education, training or leisure activities (DoH, 2005c). Work, education and leisure must therefore be considered in the assessment process. The assessment will therefore look at what is needed to keep a carer in work if that is what they wish. Perhaps this would involve a direct payment or day care or respite care. Carers should have the opportunity to discuss alternative care services and the authority should highlight the importance of equality of opportunity.

Assessments are often made on gender-based assumptions. If resources are scarce there may be a tendency (consciously or unconsciously) to base decisions on certain assumptions about who should care. Awareness of the 'hierarchy of obligation' discussed in this chapter may help to avoid sexist assumptions about what a spouse, son or daughter will do. Assessment of caring situations needs to be as free as possible from such assumptions.

In terms of anti-sexist practice, practitioners should try to identify their own assumptions and stereotypes and not base their practice on them. They should not assume that female relatives do the caring and that male relatives do little, and neither the males for the females should be given that impression. An anti-sexist approach involves men changing and doing more caring. It also involves assessors not bending over backwards to help male carers while ignoring the real needs of female carers.

Practice issues

Information relevant to practice has been threaded throughout the discussion of this chapter but some points can be emphasised and some additional points drawn out. From my own experience of practice I have come across circumstances in which considerable care, dedication and compassion are present from partners, children and relatives. On occasions neighbours and friends have provided more than one would have expected and as a result have enabled people to remain in their own homes. Sometimes carers have no longer been able to cope and needed support of one kind or another. There have also been situations where care is absent, neglect is present and abuse is suspected. A framework for practice has to be open-minded about what is going on and have the capacity to respond appropriately to the range of caring situations that exist in the community.

The community care system is bewildering to those who are encountering it for the first time. Practitioners need to provide relevant information and help guide people through it. A number of organisations (for example, Carers UK or local carers centres) provide help, advice and useful literature. Carers with particular needs can be directed to appropriate sources of information and help. Carers need to know about their right to an assessment, need to clearly know how and when it is taking place and need to be informed of the outcome of it. It is estimated that 301,000 carers in the United Kingdom move into and out of caring every year (Carers UK, 2002) and many new carers are bewildered by the complexities of the health and social care systems. Some studies have shown that often carers are not aware that they have actually been assessed (Arksey, 2002). Explaining carefully what is happening and leaving some information about the assessment and contact numbers can help to minimise this.

Carers share many concerns and facilitating their coming together is often very helpful. This requires group work and community work skills. Practitioners should find out what local caring groups exist in their area and take the time to learn what they do or ask permission to sit in on one of their meetings. They may be in a position to facilitate links between carers they know and these groups. Where there are no groups, they may be able to help set up a group. Caring is a delicate, sensitive area involving the expression of love, duty and obligation. There may also be pain, hurt and resentment. This chapter has tried to illustrate the complexity of caring and practitioners should remind themselves of this complexity and be sensitive to cues about the nature of caring relationships.

In terms of services, respite care is one of the services that carers highly appreciate. There is also a number of carers centres around the country, where face-to-face contact with a worker or other carers can help them to develop personal strategies and skills to cope with their problems. Incontinence, for example, can be very stressful for carers but local health services will usually have incontinence advisers whose practical help and advice can help make the situation much more manageable.

Heron (1998, p. 59) summarises the main areas where carers require support or service provision as break-taking, practical support, information, training in caring skills, emotional support, problem solving, effective communication, stress management and involvement in the planning and development of services. The first two relate to service provision and the rest to face-to-face work, which might involve individual work, group work or family work. A range of practitioner skills are needed when working with carers and Heron goes into this in some detail, covering groupwork theory, communication skills training, problem solving and mediation and the applicability of these to carers. She also looks at the different ways in which emotional support and information can be provided.

Later chapters in this book cover topics that are pertinent to practice with carers, in particular the chapters on social support (Chapter 6), assessment and care management (Chapter 4), user empowerment (Chapter 7) and adult abuse (Chapter 8).

Further reading

The following books (which have been drawn on in this chapter) contain thought-provoking material on caregiving within families:

The following books (which have been drawn on in this chapter) contain thought-provoking material on caregiving within families:

Finch, J. (1989) *Family Obligation and Social Change* (Cambridge: Polity Press).

Finch J. and J. Mason (1993) *Negotiating Family Responsibilities* (London: Routledge).

Nolan, M., G. Grant and J. Keady (1996) *Understanding Family Care* (Buckingham: Open University Press).

Nolan, M., Lundh, U., Grant, G. and Keady, J. (2003) *Partnerships in Family Care* (Buckingham: Open University Press).

Williams, F. (2004a) *Rethinking Families* (London: Caloustie Gulbenkian Foundation).

World Wide Web sites

A website with information on carers provided by Carers UK can be found at:: www.carersuk.org. For different parts of the United Kingdom see www.carerscotland.org, www.carerswales.org, www.carersni.org

The Department of Health has a website on carers which has useful information: www.carers.gov.uk

The Princess Royal Trust for Carers (PRTC) exists to provide information, support and practical help for carers. It has a national network of over 100 carers centres. www.carers.org

CHAPTER 3

The Shifting Boundaries of Community Care

Chapter summary

This chapter:

- Presents an overview of the key providers of community care from the formal sector.
- Discusses the way in which the boundaries between these key providers have been changing.
- Places particular emphasis on the changing boundaries between health and social care.

Introduction

Chapter 1 introduced the community care provision by social care agencies and healthcare agencies. Different agencies and large numbers of people are involved in the various aspects of community care. Service users frequently find this very confusing and require 'help through the maze', as a 1998 White Paper described it (DoH, 1998a, p. 29). Chapter 2 looked in some depth at the contribution made by the informal sector, especially the family. Box 3.1 shows the key providers of community care in the formal sector:

Box 3.1 *The formal sector – key providers of community care*

*The independent sector   *Housing providers
*Benefits and insurance providers
*Statutory social care   *Statutory healthcare

This chapter focuses on these key providers, with particular emphasis on the long-term care of older people. The list is not exhaustive. It is possible to question the composition of this list and argue, for example, that employment and education services should be present. This would especially apply if the focus of our discussion was on disabled people (Bass and Drewett, 1997).

The words 'from the cradle to the grave' are synonymous with Beveridge and everything his 1942 report stood for in terms of social welfare and healthcare. Since the early 1990s, there have been substantial boundary changes in social care and health provision that have given substance to the feeling that the 'cradle to grave' promise has been broken. The long-term care of older people is one area in which these changes have been most noticeable and this raises interesting issues of policy and practice. It is also an area in which health and social care workers frequently offer advice and guidance so it is important to be aware of the issues and engage in the debate. In this chapter, there is a particular emphasis on the boundaries between health and social care, but within the context of shifting boundaries in other sectors.

The independent sector

This sector is made up of voluntary and private organisations such as charities, user-run organisations, small family businesses and large commercial care organisations. The purchaser/provider split was brought in with the community care changes and the independent sector is on the provider side, offering services ranging from residential and day care to various aspects of home care. It provides these services through contracts with the statutory sector. The independent sector has grown considerably and its boundaries have expanded as a result of the community care changes. This has usually been at the expense of provision within the statutory sector. The shift to what is usually called the 'mixed economy of care' was a very conscious government policy decision.

Major contributors to the independent sector are charity or voluntary organisations. The voluntary sector is concerned with a broad range of issues and only a proportion of voluntary organisations are involved in community care. Those that are have had to adjust rapidly to the 'contract culture' through which services are delivered. Relations with social service and health authorities have changed in order to accommodate this. Readers may be familiar with some of the larger voluntary organisations such as Scope, Mencap, Mind and Age Concern. A further example of a large voluntary organisation working in the community care area is Turning Point. In 2006 it provided services for people with complex needs, including those affected by drug and alcohol misuse, mental health problems and those with a learning disability. It has services operating from over 200 locations and works with almost 100,000 people each year (www.turning-point.co.uk).

The emphasis on the development of a 'mixed economy of care' has encouraged the growth of the independent sector and is based on the belief that competition will improve efficiency and the resulting services will be more cost-effective than the welfare bureaucracies of the past. The reforms have meant that the statutory authorities have had a responsibility to support and stimulate the market so that a wider choice is available for users. For example, in areas such as drug and alcohol misuse and provision for people with HIV/AIDS, the majority of provision is by the independent sector, with local authorities and health authorities usually acting as funders and commissioners rather than providers. In the area of domiciliary care, there has been a very considerable increase in the growth of independent agencies and a decrease in the provision of home care provided directly by local authorities. Pollock (2004, p. 178) noted that in England in 1992, local authorities provided 98 per cent of domiciliary care services. However, by 2002 over 60 per cent of domiciliary care arranged by local authorities was provided by the independent sector (ibid.).

In the care home sector there have been similar dramatic changes. The sector ranges from very small organisations to very large companies (such as the private medical insurer, BUPA). In the residential/nursing care of older people, key shifts have been the reduction of local authority provision since the early 1980s and the rapid expansion of the independent sector, funded during the 1980s through social security payments. Between 1983 and 1996, there was a 242 per cent increase in residential and nursing home beds in the independent sector while the number of residential beds in local authority facilities fell by 43 per cent (Audit Commission, 1997, p. 10). This was a big boundary shift in a short number of years.

In her book *NHS plc: The Privatisation of Our Health Service* (2004), Pollock notes that in 1979, 16 per cent of residential care homes were in the for-profit sector and 20 per cent in the voluntary (not-for-profit) sector, leaving 64 per cent in the public sector (p. 166). By 2003, Pollock notes that 69 per cent of long-term care of older people and physically disabled people was in private for-profit homes, 14 per cent was in the voluntary sector and just 17 per cent in the public sector (ibid.). Pollock has argued that 'rather than provide care directly, the state has now largely turned long-term care over to private enterprise, and over the past two decades has created a for-profit industry worth some £6.9 billion a year' (ibid., p. 157).

The new century has brought further changes. The introduction of the minimum wage affected cost, fee and profit levels. Some independent providers saw local authority fees for publicly funded residents as unacceptably low. Some homes closed because of the anticipated costs of upgrading homes to meet national minimum standards. The 'market-place' of homes has resulted in many takeovers, mergers, sales and closures, creating instability and insecurity for residents. The result was that at the turn of the century and during the early years of the new century care home beds in the independent sector declined in numbers. The English government was generally fairly relaxed about this – arguing that people preferred to live at home and needed 'extra care housing' rather than more care home beds.

Box 3.2 The changing private sector

It is difficult to comment on the private sector because rapid changes through mergers, takeovers and auctions mean that information can be quickly out of date. At the time of writing, some of the bigger concerns in the private care home sector are BUPA, Four Seasons Healthcare, Barchester Healthcare, and the Southern Cross Group. In 2005, BUPA operated more than 290 care homes, more than 45 sites offering retirement housing and 24 hospitals (www.bupa.co.uk). As another example, the company Care UK Plc operates throughout the United Kingdom and provides health and social care solutions, including home care support and nursing and residential care home provision. It started in the late 1980s as a sheltered housing provider and was gradually changed (by its then owner Sovereign) into a business offering contracted nursing care, home care, learning disabilities and mental health provision. It has started to develop contracts with Primary Care Trusts (www.careuk.com).

Housing

In comparison with health and social care provision, housing provision has received much less attention in the discussion of community care. The choice for older people is not a stark one of staying in their own home or going into a nursing/residential home. There is a range of options in between and there could and should be more. Many services users and carers are not aware of the range of options available and need information and advice. Organisations for disabled people have often argued that 'the disabling society' prevents people from living to their full potential and housing provision is often an element of this. Houses and flats can be adapted to meet changing needs. New technology can be used in various ways to enable people to live more easily and safely in their own homes. There are various types of supported and sheltered housing schemes and some housing associations have developed a range of schemes to meet different needs. The idea of 'normalisation' (see Chapter 7), which underpins much of community care provision, emphasises the aim of integration into the community and of keeping people in socially valued environments such as ordinary housing, or as near to this as possible. Without appropriate housing, community care cannot work.

The Griffiths Report (1988) paid little attention to housing issues but *Caring for People* (DoH, 1989a, p. 3) argued that 'Community care means providing the services and support which people who are affected by problems of ageing, mental illness, mental handicap, or physical or sensory disability need to be able to live as independently as possible in their own homes, or in "homely" settings in the community'. *Caring for People* argued that suitable, good-quality housing is essential to social care packages and that 'social services authorities will need to work closely with housing authorities, housing associations and other providers of housing of all types in developing plans for a full and flexible range of housing' (ibid., p. 25).

Progress has been made towards housing being viewed as having a central and important role in community care provision. For example, The Royal Commission on Long Term Care stressed the centrality of housing, arguing that 'A larger proportion of care than now should be provided in peoples' own homes, either in the houses in which they live or in new settings which are closer to the community and which allow a greater degree of independence than traditional residential or nursing care' (Sutherland, 1999, p. 82). For example owner-occupiers who need repairs to be done or adaptations made to their houses should have access to easier ways of releasing some of the value of their houses in order to achieve this (ibid., p. 51).

There is both a need to open up mainstream housing to community care users and to provide appropriate supported housing. Supported housing, where extra help is built into the basic provisions, includes sheltered housing, hostels and shared housing. Supported housing has been used a good deal in the resettlement of people with learning disabilities or mental health problems after their discharge from hospital. Sheltered housing for older people is the largest element of supported housing, much of it provided by local authorities. Very sheltered housing is accommodation where quite a lot of personal care is also available. It has been developed by large, specialist housing associations such as Anchor and Hanover. Shared housing has also been promoted by housing associations such as the Abbeyfield Society and the Carr-Gomm Society. In the private sector as well, companies have provided both very sheltered and sheltered accommodation for owner-occupiers.

Most social service authorities have access to 'adult placement' schemes that operate on short-term or long-term bases. These schemes, which are rather like adult fostering schemes, provide a supported home environment. The boundaries of what may be regarded as residential care are shifting as different options open up.

Well-designed housing (and of course all other buildings) can increase independence and release carers from some aspects of personal care. Electronic assistive technology can also play an important role in enabling people to remain safely in their own home environment. These are sometimes called 'telecare' schemes and they usually involve some kind of sensing or surveillance technology used for monitoring vulnerable people in their own homes. In cases in which the technology identifies causes for concern, it will alert an external contact.

Increasingly the language of 'extra care' housing has been used and seen by many as an important part of future provision (DoH, 2005b). Leason (2005, p. 32) writes that it is generally 'used to describe flats and bungalows for older people that are self-contained – have a separate front door – but with some communal facilities and at least one meal provided every day. Support is usually available 24 hours a day, with personal, and sometimes even nursing care, on hand during working hours'.

Developments for the future include the idea and growth of retirement communities or villages. In the United States, these have become a key part of the housing provision for older people. The first in the United Kingdom was developed by the Joseph Rowntree Housing Trust at Hartrigg Oaks near York and was completed in 1998. The Trust is developing more initiatives. Other retirement communities are also now developing. For example, the ExtraCare Charitable Trust has developed two retirement villages (in Stoke-on-Trent and in Warrington) and has others at different stages of development.

From April 2003, local authorities in England and Wales took on responsibilities for the maintenance and development of supported accommodation arrangements. Through the 'Supporting People' programme, the government transferred a significant proportion of what had been housing benefit expenditure to local authorities so that they could commission, purchase and manage these services. The aim was to establish a more unified commissioning arrangement across a very wide range of community care and housing support schemes. Supporting People was to maintain for example, sheltered housing schemes for older people, homeless hostels, and supported accommodation for people with mental health difficulties. In the early months costs quickly spiralled and there were claims of cost-shunting by local authorities – that is, local authorities taking Supporting People money to pay for services that were previously paid for by other budgets. In 2004, the government responded by effectively capping and limiting the money available for Supporting People. Supporting People programmes started at the same time (April 2003) in Scotland and Northern Ireland. These have been similarly concerned with housing-related support services to vulnerable people and more details can be found on the web sites listed at the end of Chapter 1.

Benefits and insurance providers

For those without personal wealth, social security and welfare benefits crucially underpin the community care programme as they provide for basic essentials such as food, clothing and fuel, as well as helping with housing costs. The availability and delivery of these benefits is often critical to the sort of package of care the social worker or care manager can put together, and indeed can determine whether someone can live independently in the community at all. Thus the boundaries and linkages between the provision of social service authorities and social security provision are very important in discussions of community care.

It is well known that many benefits are not claimed by those who are eligible for them. There are various reasons for this. Potential claimants may not know about them. They may be put off by the complexity of the forms or see the system as impossible to access. They may feel too proud to claim. It is certainly a complicated and cumbersome system but it is very important for people in need of community care to have their full entitlement because poverty can only make their situation worse. If they are at home and are contributing to the cost of services, it is crucial for them to have received their full entitlement, and health and social care workers have a part to play in ensuring this happens. It is essential for practitioners to have a sound knowledge of welfare benefits so that the people they are working with can maximise their financial resources. Some published guides to benefits are listed at the end of this chapter. Box 3.3 gives a brief overview of the nature of the benefits available.

Box 3.3   An overview of welfare benefits

Welfare benefits can be divided into three basic categories, and many adults who need community care are entitled to benefits in each of the categories:

- Contributory benefits are based on national insurance contributions paid while in work. Examples of such benefits are incapacity benefit and the retirement pension.

- Means-tested benefits are paid irrespective of contributions when income and capital are less than the prescribed levels. Examples are income support and housing benefit. Under this we would include the social fund, through which it is possible to obtain community care grants (intended to promote community care by helping people move out of, or stay out of, institutional or residential care and by assisting families under exceptional pressure).
- Non-contributory benefits are paid irrespective of national insurance contributions and level of income. Examples that are especially important in relation to community care are the disability living allowance (DLA), attendance allowance (for people over 65) and carer's allowance for some carers.

It has been noted how during the 1980s the Department of Social Security met some of the costs of long-term care. Older people with limited resources could choose to go into independent homes and have their fees paid by the Department of Social Security. The expenditure in this area increased very rapidly, leading to pressure for the reforms that the NHS&CC Act 1990 introduced in relation to community care. This offered the NHS the opportunity to reduce its long-term care responsibilities and there was a significant boundary shift between the health services and the social security system.

The boundary shifted again in 1993 when social service authorities took over the lead organising and financing role. The role of the Department of Social Security (now the Department of Work and Pensions) was reduced, although of course it remained substantial. An increasing amount of local authority time was given over to ensuring that people received their full entitlement of social security benefits. Of course social service authorities realised that the more people could pay for themselves, the less drain there would be on their limited resources, and research indicated that 37 per cent of claim forms for the DLA and attendance allowance were filled in by social service authorities and allied professionals (LGA, 1997, p. 23). Social care professionals often took on this advisory task before the community care changes, but it became a greater part of their role and another aspect of the shift in boundaries. The claim forms for the DLA and attendance allowance have been lengthy, complicated and off-putting. However, for those who need considerable help if they are to continue to live in the community and maintain their independence, these benefits are crucially important. They can help towards local authority charges, help pay for private care arrangements and help with small adaptations to the home.

The Social Fund is inadequate to the task of providing flexible and quick support to enable people to live independently in the community.

The Community Care Grants under the Social Fund have a very high refusal rate and a budget that has been held very low, a state of affairs that directly affects the ability of social service authorities to help vulnerable adults to remain in the community.

For those with adequate personal resources and wealth, finding good and effective care is usually not a problem. People can buy in help for most situations, for example domestic cleaning, night sitting and nursing. Much community care is paid for by the users themselves, either through charges levied by social service authorities or by paying directly for private services. People pay from their current income, their savings, through an annuity on their property or through a private insurance scheme. With the limited cash resources of social service authorities, means-testing has resulted in many older people meeting all or part of the cost of social care themselves. They often feel quite aggrieved by this. Charging is not new but the services charged for and the amounts charged have increased a good deal since the 1990 NHS&CC Act. One aim of the community care changes was to limit expenditure. Shifting the cost of care across to service users themselves helps to achieve this aim.

One way of avoiding paying for future care out of savings and property is to take out a long-term care insurance policy. Private health insurance has become more widespread, but insurance for long-term care has been taken up more slowly. These plans can be criticised as a middle-class prerogative, available only to those who are well resourced. Take-up of them is on a small scale but they are likely to continue to figure in discussions about the funding of long-term care.

There are two types of long-term care plan. The first is known as a pre-funded plan and is for people in their forties, fifties or sixties who wish to provide for their future by paying into an insurance policy over several years. With these plans the earlier they are entered the less they are likely to cost each month. The second type is called an immediate needs plan and uses a lump sum investment to provide an immediate regular income to pay for private care.

Another example of private insurance that has developed covers home care following discharge from hospital. For example, it might help organise and fund professional short-term care at home when older patients are discharged from hospital. This is a plan for people between the ages of 50 and 79 and can be bought by the person themselves or a partner or other relative. This private insurance policy pays 75 per cent of all eligible home care fees for a stated number of days a year, depending on the level of cover chosen.

Social care

Under the NHS&CC Act 1990, social service authorities were given the lead role in the coordination of community care and the development of care management. The Act changed the financial and management structures under which care and support were provided and this involved considerable changes within social service authorities. After the implementation of the Act, people could not enter residential or nursing home care paid for by the state without an assessment coordinated by the social service authority. Hence social service authorities came to have a crucial gate-keeping role.

This was a dramatic change in the role of social service authorities and social workers. Agency and individual responsibilities increased because they had to take over some of the responsibilities of the Benefits Agency and the National Health Service. After the 1990 NHS&CC Act, social service authorities considerably reduced their own provision of residential care, focused (through eligibility criteria) on those most in need of services and took on financial assessments and charging service users to a much greater extent.

As the new system rolled out during the 1990s, budgets were overspent and social service authorities had to reduce their spending and tighten their eligibility criteria. What emerged was considerable variation in assessment, eligibility criteria and charging, leading to a lottery of care in the sense that service users in exactly the same situation could receive a very different level of services and have very different charges depending on the area in which they lived (DoH, 1998a).

With the contraction of NHS responsibilities in relation to long-term care of older people, social service authorities were subjected to considerable extra pressure due to the volume of NHS referrals. Social service authorities increased their responsibilities and costs through having a lead role but they lost much of their direct provision to the independent sector through the growth of the mixed economy. As the Audit Commission (1997, p. 15) noted, 'Placed centrally between the NHS and independent sectors, social services encounter difficulties at both these interfaces'.

A further shift of roles and boundaries came with the Community Care (Direct Payments) Act 1996, through which social service authorities could become income maintenance agencies by making direct cash payments to people entitled to care packages. In the past, cash was provided by the social security system, so here was another shift in boundaries. We saw in the previous chapter that this is an area that is expanding.

Thus there have been shifting responsibilities and shifting boundaries for social service authorities in respect of the community care changes. While the direct provision of services by them has decreased, they have taken on a lead role, increased their overall budgets and been far more involved in commissioning services from agencies in the independent sector. They have also taken on an income maintenance role through direct payments.

One can argue that the changes have been even more dramatic in the social care sector than described above. In *The Social Work Business*, John Harris (2003) writes that social work has been fundamentally changed with business thinking and practices transplanted into social work. He argues that it was the changes to community care that were central to developing this social work business and writes, 'The implementation of the NHS and Community Care Act (1990) changed fundamentally the operation of Social Services Departments and the practice of social work. It spearheaded the establishment of the social work business through two inter-related developments: marketisation and managerialism' (ibid., p. 43). We have seen how there was the purchaser–provider split, the early rule that 85 per cent of money transferred to social services should be spent on the independent sector and the explicit expectation of an increasing role for the private sector. A much tighter managerial control of what social workers did was brought in, often linked to the developing new technology. There was a shift away from the professional role, a diminution of skills, and an obsession with meeting the information needs of the new technology. Harris presents a trenchant critique of what has happened to social work and many practitioners would recognise the points he makes.

So far, consideration has been given to the contribution of the informal sector (Chapter 2), the independent sector, housing providers, benefits and insurance providers and the social care sector. We have considered the way in which their boundaries have been changing in respect of community care for older people. Consideration will now be given to the role of the health sector in community care.

Healthcare

Chapter 1 referred to some of the changing boundaries within the health service – notably the prioritisation of primary care and the increased attention given to preventive health. Also there was a considerable shift of personal care provision away from district nurses towards social service authorities (Audit Commission, 1999). We have noted earlier in this chapter the increased use of the private sector in delivering healthcare. This section concentrates on the contraction of continuing long-term care within the health service and its impact on social care services. It has been an ongoing source of tension and problems between health services and social service authorities.

The number of NHS long-stay beds was reduced by 38 per cent between 1983 and 1999 (a loss of 21,300 beds). Over the same period the number of private nursing home places increased by 38 per cent, with an increase of 141,000 beds (Sutherland, 1999, p. 34). This represents a very considerable shift of care from free NHS care to means-tested social care. The NHS's shift of emphasis towards acute care, defining everything else as 'social care', has generated a considerable amount of concern and discussion.

The case that particularly triggered changes is described in Box 3.4.

Box 3.4   Mr X and Leeds Health Authority

A 55 year old Mr X was treated at Leeds General Infirmary after a double brain haemorrhage. He was doubly incontinent and could not walk, feed himself or communicate. He also had a kidney tumour, cataracts in both eyes and suffered epileptic fits. The hospital insisted on his discharge in 1991 on the ground that nothing more could be done for him. He was then sent to a private nursing home. The cost of the nursing home was about £340 a week, and his family had to meet the shortfall of more than £6,000 a year between his income support benefits and the home's fees. Mr X's wife complained to the Health Service Commissioner, who ruled in her favour and said the hospital should compensate the family and meet all future costs of Mr X's care. The Leeds Health Authority's policy was to make no provision for continuing care at NHS expense either in hospital or in private nursing homes. However, the Commissioner ruled that someone such as Mr X, requiring full nursing care, was indeed the responsibility of the National Health Service (Health Service Commissioner, 1994).

The Health Service Commissioner (1994) selected Mr X's case from several similar complaints as an example of a general problem. He sought to ensure that the significance of his findings were not diluted by taking the unprecedented step of devoting a whole report to a single case. It had the effect he intended as the government was forced to acknowledge that the NHS had withdrawn too far from its responsibilities for long-term, continuing care.

It was clear that there were serious problems over financial responsibility, with the NHS apparently trying to redefine aspects of healthcare as social care. The government responded by issuing a guidance document in February, 1995, entitled *NHS Responsibilities for Meeting Continuing Health Care Needs* (LAC(95)5). In this guidance, patients kept the right to refuse to leave hospital for means-tested residential care. However, if they did refuse they might be sent home with a package of community care services, towards which they would have to pay. This would be 'within the options and resources available' (ibid.).

The impetus for the development of eligibility criteria for continuing care had come from the Leeds case, and LAC(95)5 was an attempt to clarify for what the health service was actually responsible in terms of continuing care. The document spelt out this responsibility only in broad terms, covering specialist clinical supervision in hospitals and nursing homes, rehabilitation, palliative healthcare, respite healthcare, community health services support and specialist healthcare support in different settings. The detail was left for health authorities to sort out in consultation at the local level. The boundaries were shifting but they were shifting in different ways at the local level.

The government of the time and the Department of Health avoided giving clear guidance on this and stressed the importance of 'local criteria'. Government ministers emphasised that it was up to doctors to decide when healthcare finished and social care started. In practice, this can often be as difficult a distinction for doctors to make as it is for anyone else. Doctors are not experts on social care and the concepts of health and social care are inherently contested and contestable. John Bowis, a government minister at the time, was given the example of somebody on a drip, doubly incontinent, relatively helpless and requiring a lot of nursing care. Even with this deliberately extreme example, he would not concur that this person was clearly on the health side of the divide (HoC, 1995, vol. 2, p. 23).

We saw in Chapter 1 that this issue was a key aspect under consideration by the Royal Commission on Long Term Care that reported in March 1999. One of its main recommendations was that all nursing and personal care costs should be paid for by the state. Thus a resident of a care home would pay for board and lodging cost only. Following on from the Royal Commission recommendations, during 2001–02 all parts of the United Kingdom introduced non-means-tested, fixed-rate contributions towards the cost of nursing care in care homes, regardless of income. However, this has not been the case in relation to personal care. It was noted in Chapter 1 that the Scottish Parliament had accepted the Royal Commission proposal while the English government and the Welsh Assembly have rejected it. In Scotland, the Community Care and Health (Scotland) Act 2002 introduced free personal and social care for people aged 65 or over. Thus in Scotland (and only in Scotland) non-means-tested payments are made by the state for personal care in care homes and for personal care in people's own homes for those assessed as requiring it.

In the rest of the United Kingdom, the issue remains contentious. Ninteen ninety-nine also saw an important legal ruling. The Court of Appeal ruled in the case of Pamela Coughlan that when somebody's need for accommodation is primarily for healthcare, the placement must be funded by the NHS. This reinforced the finding of the Health Service Commissioner in the Leeds Case of Box 3.4 by saying that NHS funding arose not only when the patient's healthcare needs were complex but also when they were substantial (Clements, 2004, p. 272). New guidance on continuing care was issued in 2001 by the Department of Health (LAC(2001)18). However, following the court ruling and the new guidance, confusion and debate continued to take place as to when a need is a health need (financed by the health service) and when it is a social care need (financed by a local authority or the individual themselves). The Health Service Ombudsman has criticised the guidance in this area (Mandelstam, 2005, p. 281) and has made important responses such as the one indicated in Box 3.5.

Box 3.5   Malcolm Pointon

Barbara Pointon had a four-year battle with the former Cambridgeshire Health Authority and South Cambridgeshire Primary Care Trust for free NHS care at home for her husband. Malcolm Pointon had a range of physical and mental health needs resulting from his Alzheimer's disease. Eventually the health ombudsman, Ann Abraham, ruled in favour of Barbara Pointon in November 2003. Following this, the Primary Care Trust accepted the recommendation and he received fully funded care in his home.

Because of situations such as the Pointon case, the Department of Health asked strategic health authorities to assess how many people were wrongly denied free continuing care between 1996 and 2002. Those families who were wrongly charged have been reimbursed. Debates on and concern about who should provide and who should pay continue and underlie some of the frustrations of practitioners in this area. The English government committed itself late in 2004 to establishing national guidelines about who is eligible for continuing care funding.

Shifting boundaries

There were three key factors underpinning some of the boundary shifts since 1990.

- The development of the mixed economy of care in social care and the marketisation within the health service.
- The demographic change in the population in relation to older people.
- The cost of long-term care and who should bear it.

The 1990 NHS&CC Act played a major role in encouraging the private sector within social care. At a local level, private domiciliary care providers grew while local authority home care services declined. Private care homes had grown in numbers through the 1980s and the 1990s with a downturn at the beginning of the new century. This opening up of the market, with the encouragement of private firms was part of the New Right philosophy that was not altered by the Labour Party after 1997.

In the same way, one can write about the marketisation of healthcare. New Labour has wanted to involve the private sector far more in health service delivery and create a 'mixed economy' of the delivery of healthcare. Important services are no longer provided by the NHS but by the private sector. There is a permeation of the NHS by private capital. One commentator who has covered the process is Allyson Pollock and she brought her argumens together in *NHS plc: The Privatisation of Our Health Service* (2004). A key point she makes is that there are now many competing providers with the private providers driven by financial incentives rather than the health needs of the population.

A second factor underpinning boundary changes is related to demographic changes within the population. With the demographic change there is a fear that the rise in the population of older people will be very expensive and unmanageable. The UK population grew throughout the twentieth century. With the improvement in life expectancy, the number of those aged 65 and over has also been growing, and since 1931 the number of older people has doubled (Sutherland, 1999, p. 13). We saw in Chapter 2 that the number of people in the United Kingdom aged 85 and over is expected to rise by 255 per cent from 1.1 million in 2000 to four million by 2051 (Wittenberg *et al.*, 2004). This is a very considerable increase but the Royal Commission on Long Term Care argued that the United Kingdom lived through its demographic 'time bomb' earlier in the twentieth century and that future projections are manageable (Sutherland, 1999).

The third factor underpinning some of the boundary shifts is the cost of long-term care and who should bear it. When setting up the welfare state a distinction was made between free services and means-tested services. The National Health Services Act 1946 introduced free care for sick people on a universal basis, regardless of their ability to pay. The National Assistance Act 1948 provided for the local care for older people who needed sheltered or residential accommodation, subject to a means test. Hence the contrasting systems of means-tested social care and free healthcare were set up at this stage. The principle of 'cradle to grave' entitlement regardless of income or assets was applied to health, education, sickness benefit and contributory benefits such as unemployment benefit and the state pension. It was not applied to long-term social care. The NHS was made responsible for sick and infirm older people, providing a free service at the point of delivery, while the long-term social care of older people became the responsibility of local government and was means-tested. Since the start, therefore, 'cradle to grave' care has never been free from payment, although many have perceived it as such. It is not the principle that has changed but rather there has been a dramatic shift in boundaries.

Long-term care of older people is expensive. This issue was tackled under the NHS&CC Act 1990 by the switch of funding to social service authorities and with the need for social workers to assess people before they could enter residential or nursing home care. As soon as 'free' health treatment was deemed to be unnecessary, people became a cost responsibility of social service authorities, which only had limited budgets. It then became crucial to decide what the dividing line was between health care treatment and social care. The former was free to the user while the second was means-tested.

Earlier in the chapter, it was noted how the number of long-term care beds provided by the NHS has declined since the 1980s. There has been a retrenchment by the NHS in this whole area. Many long-term care wards for older people (free for users) have been closed to save money. Health managers, all with their own pressures, tried to pull back from commitments on community care provision. At the local level there were disagreements over who should provide personal care, for example bathing. Health providers increasingly withdrew from this provision and social service authorities had to pick it up.

The blurred responsibilities between healthcare providers and social care providers has caused considerable tension. The overall process has involved a push from free NHS care to means-tested local authority care. The biggest shift has been the closure of hospital beds and the push towards means-tested long-term care. During the 1990s, the government's strategy seemed to be to demedicalise provision and to define it as social rather than medical care. This had the money-saving benefit of moving it out of the 'cradle to grave' NHS sector and into the means-tested social care sector.

The Royal Commission's key recommendation was that individuals should pay for their own living and housing costs (subject to means-testing) but that the state would pay for personal care costs out of general taxation. Long-term care can be financed from public finance or private finance or a mixture of both. Private sources include personal savings, housing equity, personal pensions and private insurance. Public sources include increased resources obtained through the tax system or a social insurance scheme (Harding *et al.*, 1996, p. 17). The debate goes on. We have seen how Scotland has chosen one way forward (started in 2002) and the rest of the United Kingdom has chosen another. Long-term continuing care remains one of the most important and contentious issues arising out of the community care changes of the early 1990s.

This chapter has stressed that the key providers of community care experienced a shifting of their boundaries during the late 1980s and the 1990s. Long-term care for older people has been taken as a particular example and it has been noted how there has been a cost-shunting from the NHS to social service authorities. The complexity of it all led to the setting up of a Royal Commission, resulting eventually in different outcomes in different parts of the United Kingdom. The topic is a most interesting and important area of social policy and is still very much an area of debate and dispute.

Practice issues

This chapter has discussed the need to know about and work with a variety of organisations. It has pointed to the contribution made by different agencies to community care and the importance of working with people from these agencies. The need for interdisciplinary working is discussed further in Chapter 5. Each geographical area has a different mix of provision and practitioners need to be aware of what is available in their area.

We have noted the shifting sands over when the health service will fund long-term care. This has varied a good deal and workers need to know what the current situation is in their locality. We have seen that Scotland has chosen one route. Elsewhere it is more complicated. Where someone's care needs are primarily healthcare needs, it may be possible that their care costs (whether in their own home or in a care home) could be fully funded by the NHS under continuing care eligibility criteria. Sometimes, patients and service users are not aware of this source of funding. A first task for practitioners is to find out what the published criteria are, the procedures required to access them and inform people when it is appropriate.

Patients and service users can request a continuing healthcare assessment. If they have been turned down for continuing care then the patient or a carer can ask for a review of this decision. This should freeze any immediate plans the hospital may have. If someone is being discharged to a nursing home at her or his own expense and a clinician has said that she or he only had a few months to live, a patient or carer could look at the local continuing care policy on palliative care and probably challenge this decision by saying it was the financial responsibility of the health service.

People can refuse to be discharged into a residential or nursing home, although they cannot stay in hospital indefinitely. Patients should be made aware of this so that they are not forced to go somewhere they do not want to go to in order to release a bed.

Practitioners need to be aware of and give guidance on complaints procedures within social service authorities and the NHS. They also should note the possibility of users/patients approaching the Health Service Ombudsman, who we have seen has taken a particular interest in hospital discharges and in continuing healthcare.

It is essential for all community care users to receive their full benefit entitlement, so practitioners need to be able to give sound and effective advice on this matter. Guides to benefits are included in the list below.

Funding for long-term care remains complicated and hard to understand. Practitioners therefore do require a large amount of knowledge in order to inform, advise and (where necessary) advocate. Particular emphasis has been given in this chapter to the continuing care criteria and the need for knowledge about welfare benefits, but it is important to be able to give advice in many areas. For example there is often a lack of guidance to prospective residents about choosing and paying for a care home. Useful guides for users and carers have been produced by the charity Counsel and Care (contact details below).

Further reading

There are a number of publications on welfare benefits, shifting boundaries and long-term care, including:

Child Poverty Action Group (2005) *Paying for Care Handbook*, 5th edn (London: CPAG). This is a helpful and detailed guide to services, charges and welfare benefits for adults in need of care in the community or in care homes. It covers the differences between England, Scotland and Wales.

Disability Alliance, *Disability Rights Handbook*. Produced annually, this handbook contains a detailed and comprehensive account of benefit rights and services for people with disabilities and their families. It can be purchased from the Disability Alliance, Universal House, 88–94 Wentworth Street, London, E1 7SA.

Sutherland, S. R. (Royal Commission on Long Term Care) *With Respect to Old Age* (London: Stationery Office, 1999) (main report and three volumes of evidence). This document looks fully at the issue and debates and is an obvious choice for further reading.

Pollock, A. (2004) *NHS plc: The Privatisation of Our Health Service* (London: Verso). This covers the marketisation of the health service.

World Wide Web sites

The charity Counsel and Care gives advice and information to older people and their carers. It has produced helpful guides to finding and funding care home places. Details can be obtained from its website, which is at www.counselandcare.org.uk. Its address is Counsel and Care, Twyman House, 16 Bonny Street, London, NW1 9PG.

For information on extra care housing and retirement villages visit the Housing Learning and Improvement Network web pages at www.changeagentteam.org.uk/housing.

The Joseph Rowntree Foundation is a large social policy research and development charity covering the United Kingdom. It has material relevant to most of the themes of this book, including material on the long-term care of older people. It can be found at www.jrf.org.uk.

Elderly Accommodation Counsel is a charity that gives advice and information about all forms of accommodation and care for older people. A website designed to help older people make informed decisions is at www.HousingCare.org.

CHAPTER 4

Care Management and Assessment

Chapter summary

This chapter contains:

- A description of care management.
- A description of assessment and of review within care management.
- A discussion of the assessment of need and the assessment of risk.
- An evaluation of the experience of care management.
- An introduction to community matrons and case management.

Introduction

The contribution of informal carers was the theme of Chapter 2 and the contribution of formal organisations was covered in Chapter 3. A key part of the community care strategy was that these different contributions (from the formal and informal sector) would be coordinated through care management. In *Caring for People*, there was a particular emphasis on case or care management. In situations where needs were numerous or involved significant expense, 'the Government sees considerable merit in nominating a "case manager" to take responsibility for ensuring that individuals' needs are regularly reviewed, resources are managed effectively and that each service user has a single point of contact' (DoH, 1989a, p. 21).

Caring for People and the subsequent guidance literature stated quite clearly that care management, along with assessment, were to be key elements in the provision of services. Guidance on care management emphasised that 'Care management and assessment constitutes the core business of arranging care, which underpins all other elements of community care' (DoH, 1991a, p. 7; 1991b, p. 5).

Social service authorities were required to introduce a system of care management from April 1993. However, they each did this in different ways and so a number of different types of care management and assessment systems evolved (Lewis and Glennerster, 1996; Davis *et al.*, 1997; Challis, 1999). As a result, different procedures and forms were to be found in different authorities.

The Department of Health produced quite detailed advice on care management (DoH, 1991a, 1991b), which is described as the process of tailoring services to individual needs. Seven core tasks are involved in arranging care for someone in need:

- The publication of information.
- Determining the level of assessment.
- Assessing need.
- Care planning.
- Implementing the care plan.
- Monitoring.
- Reviewing.

The last five stages are best seen as a cyclical process whereby needs are assessed, services are delivered in response to the identified needs, and the needs are then re-assessed, resulting in the possibility of a changed service response. In this way, reviewing can feed back into a re-assessment of the situation and the establishment of a new or revised care plan (DoH, 1991a, 1991b).

A case study of care management

The process of care management and the stages can be illustrated through a case study. Read first the scenario in Box 4.1.

Box 4.1   A case study

Mary Warwick lives alone in her own terraced house. There is no outstanding mortgage on the house and it is valued at about £115,000. Mary is 70 years old and her income comes from her state pension and some pension credit. She has only a few hundred pounds worth of savings. Recently, Mary has had a stroke and has been admitted to hospital. The stroke has left her with extremely restricted mobility. She has difficulty getting into and out of bed. She needs assistance getting into and out of chairs, walking and climbing stairs. The stroke has affected her left side and she cannot use her left arm or hand. She needs help with toileting, getting dressed, and the laundry. Her speech is somewhat impaired. There is concern about her ability to cope and it is felt on the ward that she may need to be admitted to a care home. However, Mary wants to return home and so the ward team make a referral to an 'intermediate care unit' (ICU). After a period in hospital, where there is some improvement of her condition, Mary is transferred to the ICU.

In the ICU, Mary has regular physiotherapy. This is hard work but Mary is motivated and makes good progress. There is a kitchen on the unit and Mary works with the occupational therapist to practice and regain her skills in this environment. A weekly multidisciplinary meeting discusses Mary's progress. This meeting involves a social worker named Janet. A date is set for a likely return home – about five weeks after joining the unit. Mary has one daughter, Sarah, who lives on her own about ten miles away and is currently working.

We shall now examine each of the seven stages of care management in order to gain an idea of what each means in relation to this situation. It has already been stressed that procedures vary in different authorities so the comments are simply to give a sense of the process.

Published information

The local authority has leaflets on care management and on direct payments and during Mary's stay in hospital and on the ICU copies are given to her and her daughter, Sarah, by the social worker, Janet. At appropriate points other published material is made available to them. This might include a leaflet on the local domiciliary care arrangements and leaflets on complaints procedures in relation to the hospital trust and the social service authority. All of this literature should be available in other languages appropriate to the local population and in braille or on tape for visually impaired service users.

Determining the level of assessment

With the introduction of the single assessment process (more details later) policy guidance has listed four types of assessment – contact, overview, specialist and comprehensive (Clements, 2004, p. 77). The staff on the intermediate care unit use the single assessment process and Janet contributes to it. She is expected to complete the contact assessment (Mary's main personal details) and the overview assessment (a more in-depth look at her situation). Other workers, for example the physiotherapist and the occupational therapist, contribute to the process by their specialist assessments.

Assessing need

Janet builds up a picture of Mary's situation through the multidisciplinary meetings. Janet gets to know Mary individually, explains her role and assesses through the single assessment process what sort of care plan or care package will be needed when Mary returns home. Janet also interviews Mary's daughter on one of her visits to the unit. Janet explains to both Mary and Sarah about care packages commissioned by the local authority and also about direct payments as possibilities for the future. Mary decides on a care package organised by the local authority. Mary goes back home for a couple of hours with the occupational therapist on the ICU, who assesses how she will manage and what difficulties there might be. A number of aids and adaptations are ordered as a result of this visit. Mary's mobility has improved quite a lot during her period on the ICU and (aided by equipment provided through the occupational therapist) it is felt that she will be able to move safely around the ground floor and use the downstairs toilet by herself. Sarah agrees to arrange for the bed to be moved downstairs at least for a period following discharge. The occupational therapist gives her views at the weekly meeting at the ICU. This informs the care plan as do the views of the physiotherapist and the nursing staff. The likely care plan is drawn up and discussed with Mary and Sarah who make some further points and suggestions. The local authority has an 'emergency alarm' service linked via the telephone to a central control room and it is agreed that this should be installed. Should Mary fall (or feel she needs help) then she can simply press a pendant around her neck and be connected to the control room, from where appropriate assistance will be arranged. A coded 'keysafe' box is also planned for installation outside the house for access if Mary cannot herself get to the door.

The local authority has eligibility criteria for community care services based upon government guidance (more details later). Janet assesses Mary in relation to these. Janet's team leader agrees with Janet that Mary falls into a category where there is a high level of need – a level of need that should be met by the local authority. Within the assessment process is a risk assessment and risk management plan and Janet follows the local authority's procedures in this area.

We saw in Chapter 3 that the cost of personal care is free in Scotland. However, outside Scotland 'personal care' services are means-tested and so people who can afford to do so pay towards the cost. Thus Janet has to undertake a financial assessment and ask Mary about any savings and clarify the ownership of the house in which she lives. This involves filling in a form with details of Mary's income and expenditure in order to work out how much she will have to pay towards any services arranged. Sometimes specialist finance officers within the local authority do this and in some authorities it may be done at a later stage following a few weeks of uncharged home care. This process is frequently experienced as intrusive and Mary may resent the questions or indeed refuse to give details.

Janet draws together the necessary paperwork that has to go to a 'panel' of the social service authority for financial approval.

Care planning

Mary wants to return home and Sarah has said she will do all she can to help her mother. Mary will need help at home so Janet has to draw up a care plan which is costed. It involves an hour's home care in the morning and half-an-hour in the evening seven days a week. The focus in the morning is on help with personal care needs early in the day. This involves:

- assistance with getting up, dressing and washing;
- assisting Mary to prepare a nutritious breakfast;
- assisting Mary prepare a snack (in advance) for tea;
- prompting for medication (if necessary).

The focus of the evening visit is to give any assistance necessary in relation to undressing, preparing for bed, and prompting for medication. The outcomes of the care plan will be expressed using the language of maximising independence and the whole emphasis of the work by the paid carers will be to work with Mary to increase her independence as much as possible. Part of the care plan involves meals on wheels being delivered every day except Wednesday and Sunday. Attendance at a day centre is to be arranged for Wednesdays. Sarah will continue her usual contact on Sundays (covering the Sunday lunch) and will call in during the week when she can. Sarah will have a word with a neighbour who Mary knows well and see if she is willing to make a contribution to helping Mary settle back into her home.

Janet formally draws up the care plan and shows it to Mary and to Sarah. Janet has outlined Mary's risks and needs, how they will be met and the outcomes that will be achieved. They agree with it and sign it. Janet gives them both a copy. This proposal and the costing is agreed by the 'panel' – made up of senior officers of the social service authority whose task is to prioritise the competing claims as their budget is limited.

Janet realises that Mary may now meet the criteria for the attendance allowance. This is a non-means-tested benefit for people who need some help with bodily functions. She takes the initiative and works with Mary and Sarah to complete the forms. The award of this benefit will help Mary to pay for some of the charges she will have to meet.

Implementing the care plan

When the money is approved, Mary is discharged and the care package is put into place. Janet has the job of ensuring that the different elements of it come together. She is on the 'purchaser' side and has to ensure that the 'providers' are 'commissioned'. 'Personal care' is usually commissioned from an agency and we saw in Chapter 3 how the 1990 NHS&CC Act had resulted in the considerable growth of private and charitable domiciliary care agencies. Janet does the work to ensure that the services are commissioned. She then needs to ensure that at the point of discharge all the services within the care plan are available and in place. A considerable amount of form-filling and work on the computer is required to put all this in place. The occupational therapist has arranged for some aids to help Mary and these have been delivered. There is liaison with the nursing staff, the occupational therapist, and Sarah about the discharge date and time.

Monitoring

Janet makes sure that the people involved in the care plan have her telephone number and asks them to call her if there are any problems. She herself checks the situation is satisfactory by appropriate telephone calls.

Review

A date for review would have been written into the care plan. This might be coordinated by Janet or by a district social worker. The review formally obtains the views of everyone concerned in order to see if the care package is appropriate or needs changing and modifying. The English *Fair Access to Care Services* says that there should be an initial review within three months of help going in or after a major change to current services. After this there should be an annual review or more frequently if the circumstances require it (DoH, 2002d, para. 60).

Mary manages satisfactorily for several months with the help provided, but during the winter she falls and later experiences a burglary, which distresses her greatly. She is increasingly frail and wonders herself if she can continue to manage living by herself. At this stage a further review is necessary. Among the options to be considered would no doubt be the possibility of:

- More support being provided for Mary at home.
- Considering 'sheltered housing' or 'extra-care' housing.
- Living with Sarah.
- Moving into a care home.

All of these have significant implications and the social worker may well have the responsibility of helping Mary and Sarah think these through. For example, if Mary moves in with Sarah, Mary will no doubt sell her house and the resulting savings may well lead to an increase in charges for any services provided. In this scenario, Sarah's needs as a carer would have to be carefully assessed and considered (see Chapter 2). Sheltered housing is an attractive option for many but ideally the planning for this needs to be done in good time. If Mary moves permanently into a care home, then her house will be sold and the proceeds used to pay for the fees of the home, depriving Mary of the opportunity of passing it on to Sarah when she dies.

Commentary

Community care is complicated and has often been described as maze or a labyrinth. The care manager has to guide the service user through a system where benefits, services and housing provision intertwine. From the Department of Health guidance (DoH, 1991a, 1991b), it is clear that the assessment of need was seen as being of central importance to the arrangements for community care and that the views of the service user should be of primary importance within these arrangements.

Janet is on the purchaser side because she is arranging the care plan. The providers include the home care service, the meal service and the day centre provision. These could be provided by the social service authority itself or (more likely now) by independent providers – this mixture is what we have referred to as the 'mixed economy of care'.

Mary's movement into an intermediate care unit gave the opportunity for careful assessment and planned discharge. The description assumes an amount of time that is often not available to social workers. We see in more detail in Chapter 5 that the reality for hospital social workers is that they often have little time to organise discharge so it is rushed and not as thorough as in this situation.

When it comes to working out a care plan, it is important to cost it. In some authorities, if the cost exceeds a certain amount it is likely that there will be pressure to enter a care home.

Assessment within care management

Section 47 of the NHS&CC Act 1990 states that, if someone appeared to be in need of community care services, then the social service authority must carry out an assessment of their needs and take this assessment into account when deciding how to meet these needs. The Department of Health described assessment as 'the cornerstone' of good quality community care (DoH, 1990) and stressed the importance of assessments being 'needs-led' (DoH, 1991b). Service users would be more involved with purchasing decisions and this would facilitate an individualised, flexible response to need (Davis *et al.*, 1997, p. 6). This was in contrast with the traditional 'service-led' assessment where practitioners were governed by the specific services their agency offered and the assessment process was dominated by whether any of these services (for example, day care, home care, meals provision) would help the service user.

The reality under the 'needs-led' rhetoric has often been that practitioners have undertaken assessments under pressure, with limited resources and with very tight eligibility criteria operating. It is the difficult job of front-line staff to manage these contradictions or conflicts in policy. Richards has written of the tension between agency-centred and user-centred objectives in assessment. She says that a user-centred approach, 'requires information gathering and provision that is meaningful to the older person and sensitive to their efforts to analyse and manage their situation' (Richards, 2000, p. 37). Often these efforts are revealed in a narrative form as the service user tells their story. If the process is dominated by agency agendas of procedures and forms then these insights can be lost with the risk of inappropriate intervention.

In the past, the more qualitative approaches to assessment were seen as the essence of professional skill. However, social workers have sometimes succumbed to the notion of assessment by ticking boxes. Increased power to managers and the routinisation of tasks has been the pattern in social work as in many of the public services – a process sometimes called 'neo-Taylorism' (Sheppard, 1995, p. 73). Sheppard notes that large areas of social care have experienced task routinisation and deskilling. Others have noted a deskilling and decline of social work, with assessment reduced to form filling in a fairly technical way (Hadley and Clough, 1996, p. 31). Such aspects of assessment are a long way from the sensitive, needs-led assessment of a person's situation. There has been and continues to be a battle as to where social work now sits on the continuum between these opposites.

In some authorities, the introduction of 'information technology' has contributed to the routinisation process. Assessments which can be fed into the computer screen are obviously quick but tend to increase the practice of using impersonalised and routinised assessments. Computers have a valuable place in welfare but they should not be used to set the agenda for community care. Practitioners can fall into the trap of thinking that doing a good assessment means filling in the form correctly or inputting the information into the computer quickly and accurately.

In the debate on the nature of assessment, a clear and helpful distinction is made by Smale *et al.* (1993) in a practice guide commissioned by the Department of Health from the National Institute of Social Work. Details can also be found in a later publication (Smale *et al.*, 2000). Smale *et al.* (1993) distinguish between the 'questioning model', the 'procedural model' and the 'exchange model'. Under the questioning model the assumption is that workers are experts in the problems and needs of people and that they exercise their knowledge and skill when making their assessment. They assess need, identify the resources required and take the follow-through action. The advantage of this for the agency is that it is relatively quick and straightforward. However, the model focuses on the dependency needs of the individual. It tends to ignore the resources actually or potentially available in the social situation and the extent to which they could be mobilised and used.

Under the procedural model, workers operate within certain agency guidelines and criteria for the allocation of scarce resources, and they are expected to gather information as a basis for judgements. 'In this the goal of assessment is to gather information to see if the client "fits", or meets, certain criteria that will "make them eligible for services"' (ibid., p. 19). Social workers have the task of identifying those who match the need defined within the categories of service available and excluding those who do not. The agenda here is really set by the agency and those who draw up the forms within the agency.

Under the exchange model, it is assumed that users, others involved and professionals all have equally valid views of the problems and can contribute to their solution. There is an exchange of information. Many people feel considerable frustration that some medical professionals assume the role of expert role on their patients, sometimes ignoring the opinions of the patients themselves. Under the exchange model, it is assumed that people are experts on themselves. Smale *et al.* argue that practitioners need expertise in the process of assessment and they list four key aspects of this (see Box 4.2).

Box 4.2 Aspects of expertise in assessment

- 'Expertise in facilitating people's attempts to articulate and so identify their own needs and clarify what they want.'
- 'Sensitivity to language, cultural, racial, and gender differences.'
- 'The ability to help people through major transitions involving loss.'
- 'The ability to negotiate and conciliate between people who have different perceptions, values, attitudes, expectations, wants and needs' (Smale *et al.*, 1993, p. 13).

Brown (1998) argues that the exchange model is the most appropriate approach when assessing the situation of lesbians and gay men. She claims that with this model 'the social worker has to work with individuals and systems involved within their own context, and has to 'hear' what is actually being said, which is often not what we might expect to hear' (ibid., p. 110). Rather than working through a long form, finding out about what people can and cannot do and then organising care and support, the approach is instead concerned with coming to an agreement about what needs doing, when it should be done and who should do it.

Chapter 2 discussed how caring relationships and commitments are negotiated over time. Practitioners need to be conscious of these negotiations and sensitive to their historical roots (Finch and Mason, 1993). The exchange model gives particular attention to the social networks of the person. A package of care is not something that can be quickly thrown together and then left. It is usually based on fragile human relationships that may need developing and nurturing. This is skilful work. The whole of Chapter 6 is devoted to the important issue of social networks.

It will be clear that Smale *et al.* are critical of questioning and procedural models that are characterised by a narrow form-filling approach. Such an approach is inconsistent with any serious vision of user involvement, user empowerment and user-led services. The job of assessment requires the skills of empathy, sensitivity, information gathering, problem solving, negotiation and judgement if the service user is to be a partner in the process.

Smale *et al.* (1993) write of the ability of the worker to create a collaborative working relationship based upon the three central skills of authenticity (or congruence), empathy and respect. These are the same sort of skills that have always been associated with social work practice and were central to social work texts of forty years ago (Truax and Carkuff, 1967). The whole book stresses the skills and competencies needed for effective care management and assessment – skills and competencies that are very much in the mainstream of traditional social work.

Mention was made in relation to the earlier case study of the single assessment process. In Scotland the process is usually known as the single shared assessment and in Wales the language of 'unified assessment' is used. Instead of having several assessments by different professional workers, the aim is to stop duplicating assessments and to share the assessment data with the other professional workers. The essential requirements of this are to place older people at the heart of assessment, to ensure care plans are produced with service users receiving a copy and to collate and share information with all of the stakeholders involved in the single assessment process. Single assessment is partly about assessment tools and 'information technology' systems. Ideally it should also be about placing older people at the centre of the assessment process. Within the single assessment process four types of assessment may be mentioned – contact, overview, specialist and comprehensive. Contact assessment is a more detailed referral and takes some basic personal information. The overview assessment is the initial screening process looking at a broad range of a person's needs. A specialist assessment focuses on specific needs and might be conducted, for example, by a specialist nurse or an occupational therapist. A comprehensive assessment would include the three assessments that have been mentioned before. It is required where there is an intensive level of support needed or, for example, where there is a possible move into a care home and it would ideally include a range of specialist assessments within it. A web site with further detail of this is given at the end of the chapter and some details of one single assessment tool are given in Box 4.3.

Box 4.3 Single assessment with 'EASYcare'

One of the single assessment tools accredited by the Department of Health is called EASYcare. It was developed at the Centre for Healthy Ageing at the University of Sheffield. It has a several pages covering the contact assessment and the overview assessment is divided into eight sections. These cover questions to the service user in:

- Seeing, hearing and communicating.
- Looking after self.
- Safety and relationships.
- Accommodation and finance.
- Looking after your health.
- Well-being.
- Memory.
- Additional personal information.

In the overview assessment there is then a section on 'planning care' which includes space to record identified needs, a risk assessment tool, an action planning sheet and a space for final comments of the service user, assessor and carer(s). Risks are clustered into five categories, with the questions that relate to each risk. The categories are mental health, physical health, loss if independence in activities of daily living, isolation/access/environment, and risk from others. Finally, there is a section on 'consent' and this relates to the sharing of personal information with others involved in and concerned about the care. A consent form is included for completion at the end of the assessment. Usually the service user will be left with the written assessment. This becomes their 'person held record' that they can show to other workers when they visit or, for example, take to hospital visits. If other workers, such as an occupational therapist, do a 'specialist assessment' then this can be added to the folder.

Weiner *et al.* (2003) were involved in a survey of the arrangements in place for health staff to work as care managers. The findings suggested that arrangements for health staff to work as care managers had not been widely developed and that there were very few authorities in which health staff worked exclusively as care managers. However, the authors did suggest that this could well change as the single assessment process got underway.

From 'needs' assessment to 'risk' assessment

The community care changes of the early 1990s raised questions about who was to be assessed and how 'need' was to be defined. If needs were defined widely and generously, then there were large resource and personnel implications. How do you 'square the circle', as Ellis (1993) put it. Lewis and Glennerster (1996) argue that the circle was squared by the Chief Inspector of Social Services in December 1992, who argued that:

- Authorities do not have a duty to assess on request, but only when they think that the person may be in need of services they provide.
- The assessment of need and the decision about which services should be provided are separate stages in the process (CI(92)34, 1992).

According to Lewis and Glennerster (1996, p. 15), 'In short, a judgment of need can be made before an assessment of need and even though a person may be judged in need the legislation does not require action to meet it. Any apprentices in circle squaring should take careful note. This is a masterpiece of the art form'.

At the end of 1993, the Audit Commission warned local authorities of the importance of establishing firm eligibility criteria for services such that there would be 'just enough people with needs to exactly use up their budget (or be prepared to adjust their budgets)' (Audit Commission, 1993, para. 15).

A considerable variation in eligibility criteria was experienced over the following decade. People with the same level of need could receive a service in one authority but not in another. This was sometimes called the 'postcode lottery'. The Department of Health in England issued some guidance to try to achieve some consistency about eligibility criteria (DoH, 2002d). This is indicated in Box 4.4.

Box 4.4   Fair Access to Care

One of the functions of a care manager is to assist with how the agency can best and most fairly use its limited resources. Service users therefore need to be categorised in terms of eligibility. The *Fair Access to Care* guidance (DoH, 2002d) was issued to try to achieve greater consistency between authorities in relation to eligibility criteria.

The guidance states that social services authorities should have a framework based on risk to independence. The information obtained from a person should be evaluated against the risks to their autonomy, their health and safety, their ability to manage daily routines, and their involvement in family and community life. These risks should be categorised into the following four bands related to levels of independence:

- Critical risk
- Substantial risk
- Moderate risk
- Low risk
  (ibid., para. 16)

Essentially the assessor is asking what would be the risks or the consequences to the person if services were not provided. The answer is then categorised into one of the above bands (Clements, 2004, p. 89). It can be seen that it is the language of risk here. This then has to be translated into need and the guidance is seen as a way of categorising need and a way of prioritising cases. The guidance does not say at which level a service should be provided and acknowledges that this will depend on the resources available to the local authority (Walker and Beckett, 2003).

The guidance mentioned in Box 4.4 is intended to help with the process of rationing finite resources on a fairer basis (between authorities) than has been the case in the past. In this way, the care manager will be very much part of the rationing process. Prioritising on 'risk' but then translating this into the language of need is clearly a key part of the guidance. It states, 'Through identifying the risks that fall within the eligibility criteria, professionals should identify eligible needs' (DoH, 2002d, para. 42). Here, one sees an example of the journey over the years from needs-assessment to risk assessment. In reality the assessment here is a risk assessment of independence rather than a needs assessment.

Risk has different aspects to it. Sometimes it is about risk to the assessor or department if something goes wrong. In relation to service users, the use of 'risk' may vary a good deal. Someone with a mental health problem may be described as 'dangerous' or 'a risk'. This language would rarely be used in relation to older people but in some circumstances they may well be described as 'at risk'.

There are two main approaches adopted by care professionals or care experts to the assessment of risk in individuals – the actuarial approach and the clinical (Parsloe, 1999, p. 13). The actuarial approach draws from the statistical data on particular populations and it is these data that provide indicators of risk from the population surveys. The clinical approach is based on the professional's knowledge of the individual's history and current behaviour and thinking. Practitioners are now often required to do a risk assessment by their agencies and often tick-box forms have been introduced in order to assist the process. One example of a tick-box tool for assessing and managing risk in relation to mental health service users was designed by Morgan (2000). Risk assessment is part of the care planning process and he writes that 'risk assessment will form one part of a comprehensive mental health assessment' (2000, pp. 22–3).

In relation to older people, Walker and Beckett argue for a holistic assessment of the whole context of older people. They write, 'Most risk assessments are done as part of a more general assessment of need. It seems very important that the interaction of need with risk be at the heart of the process' (2003, p. 48).

Reviews

There has been criticism of authorities in the past for the lack of proper review of individual cases: 'Once services are being provided, they are often not reviewed' (DoH, 1998a, p. 15). It is self-evident that care arrangements set up may not be appropriate as circumstances change and so 'reviews' are a very important part of care management. This section makes some general comments about review. For an older person, ideally the person involved in setting up the package or arranging admission to a care home will coordinate the first review. After that, social service authorities will have varying ways of organising and doing this. Sometimes a separate team may be set up to conduct the reviews. Reviews need to be determined at a time that seems appropriate to the situation. However, a review system tries to ensure a minimum of one review a year of anyone receiving a service or in a care home organised through that authority (DoH, 2002d).

People in attendance at a review will vary. A close relative or main carer would be appropriate as would be an involved paid worker. Knowledge of the situation or the paperwork may suggest other significant people such as a close friend or neighbour. Clearly, it is expected that one key participant will be the service user and their perspective will be central to the process. However, there will also be a range of care issues that need to be checked. Depending somewhat on the situation, the reviewing officer or care manager will need to go over issues such as physical and mental health, nursing care needs, medication, self-care, social contacts, finance, and the perspectives of any carers involved, whether family or friends. Issues of concern from the staff of the home or the home carers need to be considered. Clearly, if the service user is predominantly concerned with an issue such as the seating arrangements in the lounge, it can be difficult to get through the agenda. The worker has to balance the service user's concerns with the other issues that need covering. At times this can be difficult and it is important to remember that resolving what might appear to be a small matter to an outsider can bring a good deal of satisfaction to the service user and considerably enhance quality of life as they experience it.

Sometimes people involved in a review have very different needs. A busy officer in charge or matron might not feel they can afford up to an hour for a review when they have so many other matters to deal with. This might be different for a key worker who knows the resident well and is more than happy to discuss their detailed knowledge. A relative might suggest not having the resident involved for a variety of reasons – for example, the carer might feel that the service user would become very anxious about discussing finance or they might be sensitive about discussion of incontinence. Thus, some preparatory work is necessary before the review with a full reading of the file and probably telephone conversations with available interested parties to determine the best way to organise and structure the event. This preparatory work might appear to be a luxury in a busy office but in practice the effect can make the difference between a review being a paper exercise and a useful process where parties feel that issues have been listened to and addressed.

Clearly, flexibility and sensitivity are important in arranging and managing the review. Some service users might be cognitively impaired and not have the capacity to fully understand or engage in the process of the review. If it seems inappropriate for some good reason for the service user to be involved in the meeting, the reviewing officer might see them before the meeting to try to ascertain any issues or concerns. In some circumstances it may be appropriate for them to be involved for part of the meeting. It is often sensible to see the service user separately from any workers for part of the review in case they do have any concerns that they would feel unable to express in their presence.

Many reviews can be straightforward but they are important in giving time and attention to that one person. Resolving apparently small issues can significantly alter the quality of life that someone experiences. On other occasions, important issues of concern may be raised that need sensitive following up. Whatever the outcome, they are an important opportunity to give a voice to the service user and significant carers if that voice has not been heard during day-to-day activities. The review would be written up and usually sent to participants. The care plan will need to be updated and signed by the service user (in some situations it may be signed by their relative or main carer). Documentation about eligibility criteria would also usually need to be updated. A date for the next review should have been set.

The experience of care management and assessment

Reports on the introduction of care management have described the experience of front-line workers as stressful (Hadley and Clough, 1996; Lewis and Glennerster, 1996). In a study of 15 people involved in the changes Hadley and Clough painted a bleak picture, as indicated by the title of their work *Care in Chaos*. They talk of the 'massive scale' of the changes. These changes were not extensively piloted and Hadley and Clough (1996, p. 17) consider that, 'The proposals were in these ways revolutionary not evolutionary, and the belief that they would work would seem to have owed more to ideology than reason'.

In their study of assessment in relation to disabled people and their carers in the mid-1990s, Davis *et al.* (1997) explored the process of assessment in two social services authorities. They interviewed 50 disabled people and 23 carers, and observed how practitioners in six social work teams were making their assessment decisions. For most of the disabled people in Davis *et al.*'s study 'assessment' meant little. Assessment as a process that takes account of the wishes of those being assessed and where possible includes their active participation did not feature in the accounts most people gave of their contact with social workers. Davis *et al.* write that 'most people were not aware that they had a right to assessment or that their needs had been considered by a social worker' (ibid., p. 52). The authors note that peoples' lack of awareness of being a part, active or otherwise, of an assessment process was similar to the findings of other studies that have sought disabled peoples' and carers' views of community care services. Much of the practice observed in this study was based on the procedural model mentioned previously. It will be recalled that the goal of assessment under this model is to determine whether the service user meets a set of eligibility criteria. When these criteria are defined, services are effectively preallocated for generally identified needs. Social workers must then decide who matches what level of need, as defined within the categories of service available, and exclude those deemed ineligible. The requirements of form-filling and providing data for computers encouraged this model.

The researchers concluded that most of the assessments ignored the opportunity to build on strategies that disabled people and their carers had created for themselves. Much assessment was experienced as a barrier rather than a helpful way of maximising choice and independence. Some of the problems from the disabled person's point of view are summarised in Box 4.5 (Davis *et al.*, 1997).

Box 4.5   Problems with assessment

- Practitioners did not leave a name and contact number.
- With regard to paperwork, 'concern with completing items on checklists and forms blunted responsiveness to what disabled people and carers were saying and discouraged disabled people and carers from sharing more information about their situations' (Davis *et al.*, 1997, p. 58).
- Practitioners used jargon.
- There were greater problems for those whose first language was not English.
- There were long delays in social services' responses.
- There was a strict division between service users and carers – which does not match reality.

Another study that revealed great dissatisfaction with the process of assessment was Priestley's (1999) study of disabled people in Derbyshire, where there were 'delays, lack of information, poor communication, patronising attitudes, and the absence of collaborative working' (ibid., p. 94). Some disabled people and writers have argued in favour of self-assessment followed by self-management (ibid.) and aspects of these ideas have received some government support (DoH, 2000b). Care management resulting from the NHS&CC Act 1990 is generally dominated by professional practitioners, but direct payment schemes are a move in the direction of self-assessment and management. Direct payments as a method of delivering social care was given increasing government encouragement into the new century. However, it can be a big jump from being dependent on whatever services are provided by others to managing your own services, and so careful transitional planning and support may be needed. For example, people may well need help with recruitment, interviewing and employment relations (ibid.). These ideas of self-management and independent living is returned to in Chapter 7. There has also been a strong push towards 'individual budgets'

(DOH, 2005b) as a way of avoiding some of the more off-putting complications of direct payments. We return to this in Chapter 7.

There is a range of different pressures on and expectations on care managers. The contradictions within these are experienced by front line workers, who have to try to find a way through them. Some of these expectations might be listed as follows:

- Working within limited resources and therefore rationing.
- Implementing anti-oppressive practices (Thompson, 2006).
- Empowering service users.
- Carrying out 'needs-led' assessments.
- Agency expectations in relation to current government 'performance indicators' or 'targets'.
- Conducting financial assessments.
- Working in an interprofessional way.
- Encouraging greater involvement of users and carers.
- Working within a system that gives more powers to managers and routinises tasks.
- Dealing with a heavy workload within a limited period.
- Agency requirements in relation to paperwork, recording, and inputting data into the computer.

As in other areas of the public services, it is the 'street level' worker (Lipsky, 1980) who has to find a way through these contradictions and confront an array of policies with conflicting aims. It needs to be clearly appreciated that not all of these expectations can be met and that if workers are to find a way through the contradictions they have to evolve 'survival techniques'. Lipsky brought to our attention the painful reality that many workers enter employment with ideals that they then find they cannot realise. They have to 'cope' and coping strategies or survival techniques evolve. For student practitioners and newly qualified workers it is valuable to try to be conscious about these processes and explore what happens in the agency in which they are working.

One way of working within the contradictions is for care managers to paint a gloomier picture of the service user than is actually the case in order to meet a certain criterion. When this happens there is a built-in push towards pathology rather than empowerment. Here the assessment 'trick' is to portray the potential service in as 'deserving' a light as possible – according to the particular eligibility or assessment criteria. The practitioner's concern is to write down on the assessment form what people cannot do in order to achieve some sort of service for them. It can be extremely frustrating to do a full assessment and then to be told that the situation falls outside of the eligibility criteria for services to be made available. The alternative is for the practitioner to use the eligibility criteria to block the possibility of a service before the full assessment is done (Davis *et al.*, 1997, p. 49). Decisions are made to resolve the real tension between needs and resources by targeting (Lewis and Glennerster, 1996, p. 163). Only those considered to be most at risk receive an assessment (ibid.).

Case management and long-term conditions

In June 2004, the English Health Secretary announced a five-year plan (DoH, 2004a) for the future of the health services. A key part of the plan was the aim to give a priority to the personalised care and support of those people with chronic and long-term conditions – conditions that have a real and serious impact on their lives and those of their families. Long-term conditions include diabetes, asthma, arthritis, heart disease, depression, psoriasis and other skin diseases that can be controlled but not cured.

An element of this was the introduction of 'community matrons', who would have particular responsibility for that group of patients who have perhaps three or more long-term conditions and whose complex needs have meant that they have had to rely on frequent hospital stays to support them. This is under a system of 'case management', which has similarities to care management in that it has processes of assessment, planning, coordinating, managing, and reviewing the care of an individual. This will be more health led than care management and NHS and social care organisations are expected to introduce personalised case management with 'community matrons' fulfilling the lead role. The plan is that the new 'case management' will reduce the frequency of hospital stays, in part by reducing emergency admissions.

There have been considerable influences from the United States on this strategy. The pilot schemes for these within Primary Care Trusts used a model called 'Evercare', designed by the US-based company United Health, but other models may be developed. Community matrons are involved in an assessment and then the development of a personal plan. Close and constructive relations are expected with social care organisations. 'These community matrons will work with patients with complex problems to assess their needs and the support that they need and then work with the local GPs and the primary care teams to develop tailored personal plans to deliver the best possible care to them' (DoH, 2004a, para. 3.14).

Practice issues

The introduction of care management and the form it took has to be seen in the context of the ideological programme of the Conservative government and the ideas of the New Right. Sheppard (1995, p. 56) points out that care management was influenced by the strong belief in the virtues of competition, the assumption that public management was less efficient than private management and the development of a quasi-market in social care.

Some social workers were quite bemused by these changes and felt that the bureaucratisation, form-filling and financial assessments had brought an end to the traditional activities of social work. Certainly social work had changed, but it can be argued that it is continually evolving rather than ending (Payne, 1995). There were and are also some strong links to past practices, for example assessments in which the service user's views are carefully attended to are central to care management and have always been important to good practice.

The latter part of the chapter looked at a number of issues relating to the practice of assessment and care management. It is clear that there are many contradictions in the work and it is hard for practitioners to find a way through the conflicting expectations. The issue of empowerment is explored more fully in Chapter 7, but it is important to acknowledge the very real contradictions in policy that exist and have to be resolved by practitioners. Understanding what 'survival techniques' are being used allows questions to be asked about whether they are the best. Survival techniques that are at the expense of the service user should be questioned.

In doing the job myself, I have come to it believing that the service user should tell their story as they see it and that it is important to build up 'rapport' with the person. At times this is undoubtedly hard to manage alongside imparting information, gathering data for the single assessment process (sometimes leaving the documentation with them) and considering 'risks to independence' in order to decide where they fit in terms of eligibility criteria. Consciousness of the office and agency pressures might add to the feeling that not enough time is being given to doing it well. It is hard to 'bridge the divide' between agency-centred objectives and user-centred objectives (Richards, 2000).

On the positive side, since the NHS&CC Act 1990 there is undoubtedly much more opportunity to remain in the community for frail, older people if that is what they want. There is far greater flexibility of domiciliary care, more opportunities for respite, and more support for carers. Care plans have to be given to service users and signed by them and this necessarily triggers a degree of participation and involvement. There has been some welcome development of 'extra care' housing and supported housing and this has widened options. At times there can be great pressure on staff but it can also be satisfying to be part of a process that enables someone to achieve what they wish, such as remaining at home with some appropriate support.

Practitioners need to be fully aware of the procedures used in their area in relation to assessment, care management, eligibility criteria and direct payments. Service users are entitled to know how to challenge decisions and various options are open to them, each with advantages and disadvantages. Under the NHS&CC Act 1990, all social service authorities must have a complaints procedure. There is also an NHS complaints procedure. Users can contact the health service or local authority ombudsman. Grievances can be made known to local representatives such as councillors and MPs, or directly to the government. A number of community care grievances have gone through the courts to a judicial review, which is the main ground of legal challenge to local authorities (Clements, 2004).

Care management has largely been organised within social service author-ities and social service staff have usually taken the leading role. Care managers must be sensitive to the needs of carers (see Chapter 2) and the 'interweaving' of formal and informal modes of care is crucial. Care managers also need to work in partnership with other agencies involved in community care (as outlined in Chapter 3). Developments in relation to the single assessment process and the 'community matron' initiative will bring health workers much more into this work than has previously been the case. This issue of 'interprofessional working' is the subject of the following chapter.

Further reading

Walker S. and Beckett C. (2003) *Social Work Assessment and Intervention* (Lyme Regis: Russell House). This is a useful introductory and overview book on assessment and intervention. It includes child care as well as adult care but does cover areas such as assessment practice; risk assess-ment and risk management; thresholds of need and risk; and empower-ment in assessment.

Milner, J. and O'Byrne, P. (2002) *Assessment in Social Work*, 2nd edn (Basingstoke: Palgrave). This book links the theories concerned with social work practice with assessment practice.

World Wide Web site

There is a single assessment process training and learning resources website which was organised by the Centre for Policy on Ageing, on behalf of the Department of Health. There is also a link to Department of Health material on single assessment. It can be found at www.cpa.org.uk/sap

CHAPTER 5

Interprofessional Issues in Community Care

Chapter summary

This chapter:

- Describes the background to and causes of poor interprofessional working.
- Discusses attempts and initiatives to improve interprofessional working.
- Discusses interprofessional working in relation to hospital discharge.
- Provides an example of interprofessional working in the mental health field in relation to the care programme approach and care management by community mental health teams.

Introduction

Effective collaboration between agencies is a central issue in all aspects of community care not just in relation to older people, people with mental health problems and disabled people but also in areas such as adult abuse, palliative care, drug and alcohol abuse, and domestic violence. For many years there has been recognition of the need for interagency collaboration to provide a better service for users and carers. Labour's commitment after 1997 to 'joined-up solutions' to 'joined-up problems' gave this greater impetus. It has also been given a special focus with Labour's emphasis on 'partnership' working. The basic idea is frequently expressed though in a confusing variety of terms which include 'joint working', 'partnership', 'interagency collaboration', 'integrated care' and 'interprofessional working'. Glasby and Littlechild say that these different terms are a kind of shorthand to describe a way of working which is characterised by:

'• a desire to achieve benefits that could not be attained by a single agency working by itself;
- a recognition that some services are interdependent and that action in one part of the system will have a "knock-on effect" somewhere else;

- some sort of shared vision of the way forward or shared purpose' (Glasby and Littlechild, 2004, p. 7).

Loxley (1997, p. 90) argues that interprofessional collaboration is

'a device for managing and organising resources, and a technique for delivering services. To succeed practitioners, managers and policy makers require sufficient knowledge, a repertoire of relevant skills, appropriate structures for the exchange of information and resources, and processes which facilitate relationships. No one of these alone is sufficient; all are necessary.'

There is a range of general factors behind poor interprofessional working, as shown in Box 5.1.

Box 5.1   Factors behind poor interprofessional working

- A large number of organisations may be involved in providing a variety of different caring and accommodation services.
- These organisations have different structures, which makes communication at various levels difficult.
- Different organisations have different budgets and financial arrangements.
- Some of the organisations have different geographical boundaries.
- There has been weak legislative and policy guidance to promote interprofessional working.
- Workers within organisations have different backgrounds, remuneration, occupational training, culture and language, which contribute to professional barriers, mistrust, misunderstanding and disagreements.

Some writers have used the idea of 'tribes' to emphasise the differences and the problems. Dalley (1989, p. 116), for example, writes of 'tribal allegiances' that are 'not necessarily grounded in genuine differences of view but are, rather, the product of unfounded and stereotypical assumptions about those located outside the inclusive boundaries of organisations and culture'.

Some aspects of the 1990s community care changes made the situation more difficult. First, the changing boundaries described in Chapter 3 led to increased tension between agencies. Second, the community care changes deliberately created 'markets' and brought in competition between agencies. If groups and agencies are competing in a market situation then this may work against the trust needed to share information and resources and create good, effective cooperation. The concept of the purchaser/provider split within the reforms did not assist collaboration. While collaboration might be easier at the purchasing (or commissioning) level, it is more difficult at the provider level, where organisations and agencies may be in competition with one another (Lewis and Glennerster, 1996).

After Labour came to power in 1997, a commitment was given to bring down 'the Berlin Wall' that existed between health and social services (DoH, 1998d). At the end of the last century and the beginning of this, there were considerable efforts made by government to improve interprofessional and interagency working and indeed to take steps to move towards integration (Leathard, 2003). Achieving this, however, was not easy and writing in 2004 Glasby and Littlechild commented, 'For frontline workers, the need to overcome a tangle of legal, administrative and organisational obstacles in order to work effectively across service boundaries with colleagues from other professions and backgrounds is an almost daily struggle' (p. 1). In areas such as hospital discharge, continuing care, domiciliary care or rehabilitation there were considerable problems. 'For individual service users who find themselves trapped between these two large and powerful agencies, the experience is frequently one of frustration, disillusionment and despair' (ibid., p. 1).

Background to the problems

As a result of the reorganisation of both the health service and personal social services in the early 1970s, the occupational therapy service, the home help service and the social work service came under the jurisdiction of social service authorities, while the community nursing service became part of the health service. So, for example, community nursing and home care which had previously been part of the same local authority structure, were now in very separate structures. These structural barriers between service providers were superimposed on the professional barriers that existed between workers. By the mid 1970s, social work was within the realm of local government while medicine and nursing were outside of local government. These different structures and different types of accountability meant that barriers and divisions were created between the local authorities, the community nursing services, the hospital services and general practitioners.

There has been a number of attempts to bring about better collaboration. Examples of this in the 1970s and the 1980s were joint planning and joint financing. In England and Wales, joint consultative committees and joint care planning teams were established to try to achieve better cooperation. Joint financing was also introduced with the aim of stimulating and encouraging joint working. Scotland had liaison committees on a voluntary basis. However, the effectiveness of these initiatives, which were the main vehicle for promoting collaboration, was very limited. Commentators and researchers largely agree that joint planning and joint financing by the health and local authorities during the 1970s and the 1980s were weak and ineffective (Wistow and Brooks, 1988; Stockford, 1988; Lewis and Glennerster, 1996).

Given this experience, the exhortation in the 1990s for a 'seamless service' without dramatic changes seemed unrealistic. The Audit Commission (1986) was in no doubt that the situation was poor in respect of service integration and coordination. Radical reorganisation was needed and, for example, the commission recommended that for older people a single budget should be created in each area. There should be a single manager, with funds provided by the local authority and the National Health Service.

These radical suggestions were not taken up in the Griffiths Report (1988) or *Caring for People* (DoH, 1989a), both of which recommended that the structures remain the same. Thus in relation to interprofessional working there was no reorganisation of agencies but there was a call for improved coordination. Social service authorities were put in overall charge of community care and hopes were pinned on care management as a means of achieving better integration.

The exception to the above was Northern Ireland. As noted in Chapter 1, Northern Ireland had combined services under four ministerially appointed health and social services boards, set up in 1973 and responsible for both health and social services. The House of Commons Health Committee looked to the integrated service of Northern Ireland as a possible model for the rest of the United Kingdom, arguing that 'we found much to admire in the integrated model adopted in Northern Ireland' (HoC, 1999, para. 68).

In the absence of structural reorganisation, another way forward in the early 1990s would have been to establish strong financial inducements and a powerful legal mandate to encourage cooperation. Some efforts were made in this direction but they were limited. In 1993, the payment of the Special Transitional Grant was made conditional on health authorities and social service authorities establishing local agreements on the placement of people in nursing home beds and on hospital discharge arrangements. On the legal side, Section 46 of the NHS&CC Act 1990 required local authorities to consult a range of organisations when formulating and reviewing community care plans. The Act also imposed a duty on social service authorities to notify the local housing authority and appropriate health services and invite them to assist in assessment when a potential housing or health need was identified. However, no obligation was imposed on the housing authorities or on the health services actually to give assistance. This legal mandate clearly could have been stronger. So the community care changes of the early 1990s did not address the reorganisation of services or impose a powerful legal mandate. As before, the need remained to make structures work effectively and efficiently together so that users had the best possible service and funders the best possible value for money.

Chapter 3 noted that the strategy in the early 1990s seemed to be to demedicalise provision and define many activities as social care rather than medical care. Hence there was cost-shunting from the free health services to the means-tested social services, which provided the potential for increased tension between workers in the health and social care sectors. Chapter 3 indicated that the health authorities redefined their areas of responsibility for continuing care to such an extent that an alarmed government took steps to prevent it from going any further. At the point of the interface between workers at the bottom of their organisational hierarchy, it was not surprising that it was hard to make interprofessional practice work. What was surprising was that workers often did overcome many of the structural problems, frequently because of their commitment to a public service ethos.

In their study of the implementation of the 1990 community care legislation by five local authorities, Lewis and Glennerster (1996, p. 167) state that 'action to achieve collaboration in community care has taken a variety of forms in the 1990s. Authorities were faced with the question of what to do about the elaborate 1980s joint planning machinery.' Lewis and Glennerster argue that it was not abolished but 'reworked in relation to the emergence of the purchaser-provider splits and renamed "joint commissioning"' (ibid., p. 167). Joint commissioning was defined as 'the process in which two or more commissioning agencies act together to coordinate their commissioning, taking joint responsibility for translating strategy into action' (DoH, 1995b, p. 2). While the district health authorities and social service authorities were central players in joint commissioning, housing departments, family health service authorities, GPs, GP fundholders and other providers of health and social care could also be involved. Joint commissioning was seen as a more productive way forward than joint planning and joint financing. Old structures of joint planning still existed but had been modified and revamped in the 1990s (Lewis and Glennerster, 1996).

Joint commissioning was seen as a way of collectively taking community care forward after the failure of joint planning (Poxton, 1996; Leathard, 1997). According to Poxton (1996, p. 143),

'In essence, joint commissioning seeks to bring together some or all of the commissioning functions of a number of different agencies, usually with health and social services at the core. It may be focused on a particular user group, on a range of services, on a geographical locality, or even on the needs of a particular individual.'

However, Lewis and Glennerster (1996, p. 186) gave a rather bleak assessment that without drastic action 'The fundamental conflicts between agencies that are financed separately, administered separately, staffed by different professions and run within different statutory frameworks are so great that no joint commissioning or joint planning has much hope of succeeding'.

Partnership and integrated care

The achievement of better inter-agency working was a priority for the Labour government after its election in 1997. It stressed this in a variety of documents, initiatives and proposals, for example 'The Government has made it one of its top priorities since coming to office to bring down the "Berlin Wall" that can divide health and social services, and to create a system of integrated care that puts users at the centre of service provision' (DoH, 1998a, para. 6.5). There were no proposals for major structural change in the sense of integrating services within one organisation. 'Major structural change is not the answer' (DoH, 1998c, p. 5). Clearly, some changes were taking place in some parts of the country. Changes such as:

- social work staff seconded into health service teams to become part of a multidisciplinary team;
- locating social work teams in health centres;
- appointing nurses or seconding nurses to social work teams.

These types of changes were encouraged and continued but further steps were soon on the agenda that were certainly moving in the direction of structural change. These changes saw movement towards pooled budgets, lead commissioning and integrated provision through enactment of the necessary legislation as indicated in Box 5.2.

Box 5.2   Removing legal obstacles

The Health Act 1999 for England and Wales removed legal obstacles to joint working and gave both parties new powers to work together. This was under Section 31 of this Act and hence the agreements are sometimes called Section 31 agreements. This included:

- Pooled budgets: health and social services can put money into a single dedicated budget to fund a wide range of care services.
- Lead commissioning: either the health authority or the local authority can take the lead in commissioning services on behalf of both.
- Integrated providers: health authorities and local authorities can merge their services to deliver a one-stop package of care.

Similar arrangements were made possible in Scotland under provisions of the Community Care and Health (Scotland) Act 2002.

Thus structures developed that often facilitated better and easier communication between different professional workers. This was an important part of the process. Another has been workers seeing joint working much more as a part of the job that they themselves do. A number of parallel changes have linked into the more structural changes and sometimes contributed to this changing self-definition. Changes such as the move towards a single assessment process have contributed towards this self-perception as have the growing number of 'rapid response' teams to prevent hospital admissions, comprising both nursing and social work staff. A third example might be the creation of joint stores (social services and health) of equipment, which service users might need to remain in the community. It is rather early to establish the overall impact of these various changes but it is certainly true that a great deal of emphasis has been put on 'partnership working'. As Dowling *et al.* wrote, 'The message is clear: the pressure to collaborate and join together in partnership is overwhelming. Partnership is no longer simply an option; it is a requirement' (2004, p. 309). The English Green Paper (DoH, 2005b) very much continued to envisage partnerships helping towards more integrated care. In the later White Paper (DoH, 2006) quite a number of measures on joint working were proposed including the alignment of NHS and local government financial cycles, joined-up performance management and joint teams to support people with the most complex conditions.

In Scotland, there has been a similar emphasis on partnership but some differences of approach. In 1999, the Joint Future Group for Community Care was set up by the Health and Community Care Minister. A key aim was to promote the debate about promoting integrated community care based on an understanding and agreement that joint working between the NHS and local authorities could be improved. Local partnerships have been central to community care developments in Scotland. The Scottish Community Care and Health Act 2002 enabled and expected local partners to delegate functions and pool budgets (Hudson, 2005). Hudson writes that 'All local partnerships now have to produce extended local partnership agreements for all community care groups, showing progress made against the indicators contained in the joint performance information and assessment framework' (ibid., p. 37).

Particular services that have been encouraged in Scotland through this process are:

- Rapid response services to keep people out of hospital.
- Intensive home care.
- Joint equipment services.
- Simple shared assessment.
- Joint servicing and joint management of services.
- Integrated community care services.

In the document *Better Services for Older People: Framework for Joint Services* (Scottish Executive, 2005), the direction has been given to partnerships to focus on improved outcomes for individuals and their carers as part of a way of re-invigorating the Joint Future Agenda. In the Foreword to this document it says,

> 'Joint Future has come a long way in the past three years. Local social care, health care and housing partners have developed more mature and open ways of working together and have set in place many structures and systems such as joint committees and single assessment. The time is right to move on – to look much more at how we can translate that into better outcomes for people and their carers' (ibid., p. 5).

Hospital discharge – at the 'fault line' of interprofessional working

One of the issues that has always been problematic in relation to inter-agency collaboration is hospital discharge. In an overview of the topic published in 2003, Glasby wrote, 'Although inter-agency collaboration is often complex and problematic, it is hospital discharge rather than any other issue which generates the most tension and causes the most difficulties for the service users and workers involved' (2003, p. 1). He described it as 'a fundamental fault line between two very different services' (ibid.). In the conclusion to his study, he noted the opinion of the House of Commons Health Committee (HoC, 2002) that there needed to be structural change involving the integration of the health and social care system. He also took this view, arguing that, 'major structural change is the only way to achieve successful partnership working and to improve the experiences of older people and other service users discharged from NHS hospitals to health and social care in the community' (Glasby, 2003, p. 131).

In England, the strategy that was designed to deal with this 'fault line' was the Community Care (Delayed Discharge) Act 2003. This set out to deal with what had often been called in the past the problem of 'bed-blockers'. This Act introduced a system of reimbursement by social services to the relevant NHS body for delays caused solely by the failure to provide timely assessment and/or social care services. The claimed intention was not that social service should make payments to the NHS, but to provide an incentive to invest in an extended range of services that prevent delays from occurring in the first place. It linked into the development of intermediate care facilities, more community based care arrangements and the single assessment process – all of which had a strong emphasis on interprofessional working.

Under the 2003 legislation, NHS bodies have to make two notifications to social services departments in order to trigger a claim for reimbursement. The first (a Section 2 Assessment Notification) gives notice of the patient's possible need for services on discharge. Following this notification, social services departments have a minimum period of three days to carry out an assessment and arrange services. The second notification is a Section 5 Discharge Notification and this gives notice of the day on which it is proposed that the patient is to be discharged. Liability for reimbursement begins on the day after the minimum three-day period (Section 2) or the day after the proposed discharge date (Section 5), whichever is the later.

A report on the first six months of this experience by the Commission for Social Care Inspection concluded that, 'The early indications from the statistics are that the reimbursement policy has contributed positively to the downward trend in discharge delays that had already begun' (CSCI, 2004, p. 3). Also on the positive side it argued that it had 'brought health and social services together rather than pulled them apart' (ibid., p. 47).

However, on the negative side some of the aspects of concern identified by the Commission were:

- 'anecdotal evidence of people being pressurised to leave hospital prematurely without proper arrangements for their continuing support' (ibid., p. 3).
- in some councils up to a third of older people needing social services support on leaving hospital were moving directly into residential care or nursing homes. The report comments that, 'Pressures to free up

beds should not, in turn, pressurise older people into making long-term decisions about where they live' (ibid., p. 5).

- 'There was also some evidence from our sample of cases of a high number of readmissions within a few months of discharge, over 50% in one locality' (ibid., p. 25).

A later follow-up report (CSCI, 2005) charted the experience of these same older people nine months after they were discharged from hospital. It showed that where people had been moved directly into care homes from hospital, this was likely to be permanent. While for some it was an acceptable move, for others it was 'a hurried decision that had come to be regretted' (ibid., p. 6).

At the time of writing, it is too early to properly evaluate this attempt to deal with the problem. Drawing on a comprehensive review of the literature on delayed discharges, Glasby *et al.* (2004) note the complexity of the factors causing delayed discharge. A large number of studies indicate the need for more rehabilitation services, an issue that has been addressed by policies and funding. Many studies identify internal hospital factors as a key issue. The writers note there is a great diversity in the causes of delayed discharge with these varying substantially from area to area. However, the main legislative policy response has been the 2003 Community Care Delayed Discharges Act. Glasby *et al.* conclude, 'it is difficult to avoid the conclusion that social care is "carrying the can" for a problem not of its own making and that current policy has dramatically oversimplified a much more complex problem' (Glasby *et al.* 2004).

Mental health as an illustration of issues in interprofessional working

It was mentioned at the start of this chapter that interprofessional working is an important aspect of every area of community care. In order to analyse this issue we shall look at mental health provision. This area has sometimes resembled a battleground between health and social care, and a number of reports indicated that poor inter-agency working is a real problem in the mental health services (Audit Commission, 1994; Ritchie *et al.*, 1994; Utting, 1994). In addition to the problems outlined earlier in the chapter, there is also the historical domination by psychiatrists, often leading to tensions over leadership and control.

Over the past forty years, there has been a gradual but substantial change from hospital-based to community-based mental health services.

The management of these services has caused considerable problems and there has at times been strong public criticism of the policy. Media campaigns have repeatedly asserted that community care has failed in the case of mental health service users. There have been several inquiries resulting in policy changes – principally the development of the care programme approach (CPA) and the further development of community mental health teams (CMHTs).

People with mental health problems have a diversity of needs that span a variety of agencies and workers. These agencies have different structures, managements and cultures. Professional workers are trained on different courses, often in different institutions. There has been relatively little joint training. The segregation of professional training and job structures allows stereotypes of workers in groups to develop. These divisions can impede the delivery of effective service. This section looks first at CPAs and care management, both of which are concerned with improving interprofessional working, and then at the work of CMHTs.

The care programme approach and care management

During the 1960s and the 1970s, there were several inquiries into hospital scandals, usually involving patients being badly treated by abusive staff in an abusive care regime. During the 1980s and especially the 1990s, further inquiries often raised profound anxiety about the policy and practice of community care. In 1988 came *The Report of the Committee of Inquiry into the Care and Aftercare of Miss Sharon Campbell*, who had knifed to death her former social worker, Isabel Schwarz, at Bexley Hospital (Spokes *et al.*, 1988). The Campbell Inquiry recommendations led to the care programme approach (CPA)

One of the main reasons for introducing the CPA was to try to improve interprofessional communication and coordination. Interprofessional work was viewed as central to achieving a better service and the CPA was seen as a means of bringing this about. Health authorities were required to develop a CPA for people with a severe mental illness (people referred to specialist psychiatric services). The approach required health authorities, in collaboration with social service authorities, to design and implement arrangements for treating service users in the community and ensuring that they received the necessary care. Under CPA, the needs of each patient, in relation both to continuing health care and to social care, were assessed before discharge. Each patient had a key worker whose task it was to keep in touch with the patient in the community. The essential elements of the CPA are shown in Box 5.3.

Box 5.3   The four main elements of the care programme approach

- 'Systematic arrangements for assessing the health and social needs of people accepted into specialist mental health services.
- The formulation of a care plan which identifies the health and social care required from a variety of providers.
- The appointment of a key-worker to keep in close touch with the service-user and to monitor and coordinate care.
- Regular review and, where necessary, agreed changes in the care plan' (NHSE/SSI, 1999, para. 4).

The interprofessional aspect of CPA is illustrated by the following:

'Specialist psychiatric services are provided by a multi-disciplinary team of individuals each with his or her particular skills and experience. It is this dimension that makes inter-agency working so crucial, particularly for severely mentally ill people. The multi-disciplinary CPA can only function where all those in the team work effectively together, for the good of the patient' (DoH, 1995, p. 14).

A somewhat strange policy development in community care was the simultaneous introduction of two separate but similar systems of caring for people with mental health problems, namely the care management and the care programme approach. Care management and CPA were similar in that they both included the same core tasks of assessment, planning, implementation and review. They were different in that CPA included a key worker idea (providing direct support and counselling) in contrast to a care manager, who organised and coordinated support. They were also different in that CPA was health-led and care management was local authority-led (DoH, 1990). Reports during the 1990s indicated that there was continuous confusion about these different procedures (North et al., 1993; Audit Commission, 1994; DoH, 1994). Onyett writes, 'In practice, much confusion surrounded the relationship of the CPA to care management' (2003, p. 37).

In 1996, the Department of Health issued a publication entitled *Building Bridges*, which was a guide to arrangements for interagency work in the care and protection of severely mentally ill people (DoH, 1995a). It outlined the roles of agencies involved in caring for mentally ill people and stressed that 'The CPA is the cornerstone of the Government's mental health policy' (ibid., p. 45). The Department of Health provided no rationale for having two similar case-planning approaches with different titles, simply arguing that, 'If properly implemented, multi-disciplinary assessment will ensure that the duty to make a community care assessment is fully discharged as part of the CPA, and there should not be a need for separate assessments' (ibid., p. 15). It was argued that the two systems could be integrated by treating the CPA as a specialist variant of care management for people with mental health problems (ibid., p. 56). After its election in 1997, the Labour government continued to stress the importance of care management and the CPA for the delivery of effective treatment and care (DoH, 1998c). Some form of integration was achieved in guidance in 1999 (NHSE/SSI, 1999).

Case study – Christopher Clunis

Building Bridges (DoH, 1995a), referred to above, was produced in response to the Ritchie Report on the murder of Jonathan Zito by Christopher Clunis (Ritchie *et al.*, 1994). This was probably the best-known mental health inquiry report of the 1990s and it filled 130 pages with 78 detailed recommendations. Recurring themes in the report were the missed opportunities and failure of communication. For example:

- A large number of psychiatrists and social workers had been temporarily responsible for Clunis's care over six years. At one time he had asked to see a psychiatrist in order to review the medication he was on, but he had not been seen for 13 months.
- A GP whom Clunis had visited had struck him off his list because he was abusive and threatening.
- Over several years there had been a number of warning signs of Clunis's tendency for violence, including the use of knives in some potentially fatal incidents before the actual incident with Jonathan Zito. For example, Clunis had stabbed a fellow hostel inmate and had been charged with causing grievous bodily harm with intent. The police had made little effort to trace the victim before the case came to court and no effort to obtain independent evidence. The case was dropped.
- A number of agencies had failed to pass on information about Clunis's acts of violence.
- There had been both ambiguous definition and ambiguous allocation of responsibilities within the mental health services.
- The various agencies involved had not attempted to involve Clunis's family in his care, despite the fact that his sister in particular had been in reasonably regular contact with him.

The Ritchie Report concluded that Clunis' care was 'a catalogue of failure and missed opportunity' (ibid., p. 105) from 1987 until 1992. Over this period, Clunis had stayed in various psychiatric units and hostels for the homeless, unable to care for himself because of his mental illness. At various points there had been both the opportunity and the legal power to do something, but nothing had been done. Clunis had repeatedly fallen through the nets of care, with overstretched agencies apparently having neither the will nor the determination to work together in his interests. It was clear that there should have been better communication and coordination between agencies and a better working partnership with Clunis's family.

Another clear theme of the report was that the problem could not be blamed on a lack of resources. In his introduction to *Building Bridges* (part of the government's response to the Ritchie Report) the Parliamentary Under Secretary stated that:

> 'People who are severely mentally ill are likely to be receiving health and social care from a number of different agencies in the statutory, voluntary and independent sectors. All those involved need to work closely together to ensure that their combined resources are used to best effect and, most importantly, that vulnerable patients do not fall victim to gaps in service provision. Links between health and social services are of course vital, but they are by no means the only ones which need to be made.' (DoH, 1995)

Building Bridges highlighted the need for better sharing of relevant information and for a better coordination of services: 'The key principle underlying good community care for mentally ill people is that caring for this client group is not the job of one agency alone, just as it is not the responsibility of one professional group alone' (ibid., p. 26). While it was recognised that service providers were increasingly working in teams, what was left unresolved were questions of accountability and responsibility among practitioners working in multidisciplinary teams. These ambiguities were long-standing and contributed to ambivalence about multidisciplinary teams among professional practitioners (Galvin and McCarthy, 1994). The next section looks at this in more detail.

Community Mental Health Teams

According to Wells, 'Community Mental Health Teams (CMHT) have been identified as the vehicle through which mental health care in the community, encapsulated in the "Care Programme Approach" should be delivered' (Wells, 1997, p. 333). Two mechanisms (CPAs and CMHTs) are in place to help make multidisciplinary working effective within the mental health field. Government guidance has also stressed the import-ance of teams: 'Specialist services working in hospitals and the community are increasingly working in teams. This is recognised as the most effective way of delivering multi-disciplinary, flexible services which the principles outlined above demand' (DoH, 1995a, p. 35). Simpson *et al.* wrote that, 'The effective discharge of individual CPA responsibilities can only occur in the context of a "well-functioning team" under good leadership' (2003, p. 497).

The CMHTs are multidisciplinary in composition and are responsible for coordinating and delivering a specialised level of community-based care for defined populations (Carpenter *et al.*, 2003). Carpenter *et al.* write, 'Teams in England include psychiatric nurses, psychologists, occupational therapists, and psychiatrists who are employed by health trusts and social workers seconded by local authority social services departments' (p. 1082). It is argued that integration between health and social services characterise the future of mental health services (ibid.). Policy guidance asserts that, 'CMHTs function best as discrete specialist teams comprising health and social care staff under single management (DoH, 2002c, p. 18).

A frequent criticism of CMHTs is that the role of team members is not clear. Being members of two groups – a professional discipline and an interdisciplinary team – they can be torn in two directions. Onyett *et al.* suggest that,

'It might therefore be predicted that the ideal conditions for team membership would be where a positive sense of belonging to the team can exist alongside continued professional identification. This is most likely to occur when the discipline has a clear and valued role within the team, which in turn requires that the team itself has a clear role.' (1995, p. 22)

An interesting debate has emerged as to whether CMHTs can overcome all the problems and bring about effective multidisciplinary working practices. Perhaps the strongest argument against their ability to do this has come from Galvin and McCarthy (1994), who argue that they are 'fatally flawed' and that the provision they offer is unfocused, inefficient and of poor quality. They argue that this is an inadequate model and that alternative models of mental health service provision are needed. A main cause of the problem is the complexity of the tasks the teams have to tackle which they are poorly equipped to handle. Too much has been expected of them.

Galvin and McCarthy argue that the CMHTs have an overambitious agenda; that the need for CMHTs is assumed rather than argued for; that issues of accountability and responsibility are fudged both within the CMHT and in relation to external management. Teams are left to cope with problems that are beyond them – differences of history, policy, mechanism and goals. 'Teams are expected to resolve complex national issues such as the status of individual members, professional training, levels of competence, legal status, entitlement to practice autonomously, and the functional inter-relationships between professional groups without any definitive central policies or even guidance' (ibid., p. 164). These issues are far too significant and distant to be resolved by improving the processes locally within the teams. CMHTs appear as though they are tackling the community mental health agenda but they are not. 'CMHTs are attractive because they provide a convenient means of pushing conflicts down the system' (ibid., p. 165). Galvin and McCarthy stress the importance of not dodging issues that arise higher up the system.

The views propounded by Galvin and McCarthy are just one perspective on the issue and they are at one end of a continuum. The consensus however is very much in favour of CMHTs as a key means of delivering community mental health care. Onyett and Ford (1996), for example, do not accept that the concept of multidisciplinary teamworking is inherently flawed and they make a convincing case for its continuation.

Onyett argues that CMHTs, far from being a failed project, are a key vehicle for collaborative care but that attention needs to be given to questions of implementation (Onyett, 1997). He notes that the develop-ment of case management was a US social policy measure to improve targeting, followed in the United Kingdom by CPA and care management. He argues that there were disappointing outcomes in case management and keyworking when they operated as a means of service coordination and follow-up outside a multidisciplinary team (ibid., p. 264). Thus CPAs need CMHTs in order to work effectively.

In the United States, research indicates that community mental health teams and centres failed to prioritise services for people with severe and long-term mental health problems until there was a switch to an emphasis on case management coordination (Onyett *et al.*, 1994). Similarly in the United Kingdom, CMHTs have been criticised for neglecting people with severe mental heath problems (Patmore and Weaver, 1991), and case manage-ment coordination (CPA and care management) has been developed to help address this issue.

Guidance on CPA and care management has stressed the importance of the multidisciplinary team working for people with severe, long-term mental health problems. The main vehicle for multidisciplinary team working is the CMHT and thus it has been proposed that CPA and care manage-ment be integrated within CMHTs. Other important elements for effective interprofessional working are a joint strategy, good information sharing, joint training and management support for a culture of interprofessional communication (Hancock and Villeneau, 1997, p. 33).

Practice issues

On the ground it can sometimes feel as though there is a great deal of personal conflict between different professional workers, but this is usually symptomatic of underlying structural and organisational problems. It is important for practitioners to keep this in mind. It is too easy to fall into the trap of blaming the woman/man in the agency around the corner for things that are going wrong rather than understanding and appreciating the wider context. There is a need for an understanding and an analysis at an individual, organizational and structural level (Glasby, 2003).

The reasons for the difficulties are many and complex so there are no easy solutions. There is a need for changes at all levels – political, organisational, managerial and educational. However this should not be an excuse for practitioners to do nothing. It is worth reflecting on the following quotation from the Brazilian educationalist Paulo Freire: 'How can I enter dialogue if I always project ignorance on to others and never perceive my own?' (Freire, 1972, p. 63).

A variety of initiatives can be taken at the personal and local level. Freire's comment suggests the value of finding out about the work and values of other workers. It is all too easy to become embroiled in one's own speciality and lose one's sense of a shared aim. Just as GPs and community nurses are not experts on social care, neither are social workers experts on health and medical care. There is a need for mutual respect, and for listening to and learning from others' experiences and expertise.

In an overview of *The Health and Social Care Divide*, Glasby and Littlechild do not minimise the difficulties which remain, 'Across a range of services, different cultures, policies, agendas, funding priorities, administrative systems and legal requirements all have the potential to make day-to-day experience of interagency collaboration extremely frustrating, time-consuming and, all too often, unsuccessful' (2004, p. 147). Thus there are organisational and structural issues that make it very difficult for practitioners.

Interprofessional working is increasingly taking place in teams. This chapter has discussed some of the concerns about and debates on this way of working. It has particularly indicated that when working in such teams practitioners may feel pulled in different directions. Most obviously they may feel different obligations and accountability to their professional team and group than they do to the multidisciplinary group in which they are working. This is a common problem that needs to be talked about and worked through.

The growing interest in interprofessional education led to the formation in 1987 of the Centre for the Advancement of Interprofessional Education in Primary Health and Community Care (CAIPE). CAIPE was the first organisation to promote development, practice and research in shared learning. It has continued to promote shared learning and provides support for those offering it. It collects and disseminates information, helps with networking, organises conferences, commissions and conducts research and publishes a twice-yearly bulletin. Further information can be obtained from its website which is given below.

Further reading

Leathard, A. (ed.) (2003) *Interprofessional Collaboration* (Hove: Brunner-Routledge). A selection of chapters on aspects of interprofessional collaboration.

Glasby, J. and Littlechild, R. (2004) *The Health and Social Care Divide* (Bristol: Policy Press). The aim of the book (which uses several case studies) is to help practitioners to work more effectively together.

Onyett, S. (2003) *Teamworking in Mental Health* (Basingstoke: Palgrave). This is a guide to aspects of teamwork in the field of mental health.

World Wide Web sites

The Sainsbury Centre for Mental Health has information on mental health services at http://www.scmh.org.uk

The Centre for the Advancement of Interprofessional Education in Primary Health and Community Care (CAIPE) has a website at www.caipe.org.uk

The website of the Integrated Care Network helps care organisations work together and explores a range of partnership topics. It can be found at www.integratedcarenetwork.gov.uk

CHAPTER 6

Social Support and Community Care

Chapter summary

This chapter:

- Discusses the concepts and links between community, social support, social capital and health and the significance of these for practitioners.
- Considers the ways in which practitioners can develop partnerships in their work and the importance of transitions within community care.
- Explains what networks are, how they can be measured, their different types and how they can be worked with in community care practice.

Introduction

Chapter 2 explored the role of carers in community care and introduced the idea of interweaving informal and formal care. Chapter 4 emphasised the importance of this within care management and of the need to have good knowledge of the support being given by informal carers. This chapter develops this discussion by looking at the concepts of social support, social capital and social networks. It argues that health and social care practitioners need to work with support networks in a sensitive and constructive way.

This chapter draws on a tradition of intervention that involves identifying, supporting, developing and extending the support networks of the service user. This tradition has sometimes been called the ecological perspective. It emphasises the skills required for assessing networks and working with them in a sensitive way. Support systems and support networks vary according to divisions of class, gender, sexuality, race and age. Skills in and knowledge of anti-oppressive practice are important in these situations because it is important not to put more pressure on women to care or reinforce the myth that black people and ethnic minority groups 'look after their own'. Thus a commitment to redress the inequalities and discrimination that occur within services and within society must be a part of this approach.

The term community care has 'community' within it and this is a much contested term. One author identified 94 different definitions (Hillery, 1955). 'Community' can be used to describe a group of people in the same situation (for example, the elderly residents of a residential home) or people with something in common (for example, the gay community). Probably still the most common use of the word relates to geographical area.

In the early 1980s, government publications moved from talking about care *in* the community to care *by* the community and this distinction was incorporated into official policy (DHSS, 1981, p. 3). Neither care *by* the community nor care *in* the community is really a tenable choice. The aspiration should be towards care *with* the community (Froland *et al.*, 1981, p. 165). Collins and Pancoast (1976, p. 178) believe that 'care *with* the community is the most viable and productive direction for the future development of human services'. Both this chapter and the next discuss some ways in which this can be done.

Social support and health outcomes

Cassel (1974) and Cobb (1976) brought together evidence that the health outcomes of people who experience high levels of stress vary according to level of support or access to support. Caplan (1974a, 1974b) is well known for developing and furthering these ideas in the mental health field. This early work led to many studies of and action projects on the health-protecting functions of social support. There is now a very considerable body of literature on the subject (for example, Cohen and Syme, 1985; Taylor, 1993; Ell, 1996; Cooper *et al.*, 1999; Kawachi and Berkman, 2001). According to the White Paper *Saving Lives: Our Healthier Nation*, 'There is increasing evidence, including from the World Health Organization, that having strong social networks benefits health' (DoH, 1999b, para. 10.21). David Putnam puts it simply that, 'Social networks help you stay healthy' (2000, p. 331).

In order to illustrate this, let us use a fictional example of an elderly couple, Mr and Mrs McDonald. They are both in their eighties and have lived together for 55 years. Mr McDonald dies suddenly of a heart attack. Because of their long and close relationship this is a very serious life event for Mrs McDonald. Her bereavement may result in serious emotional distress and illness, a situation that is familiar to workers with elderly people and is shown diagrammatically in Figure 6.1.

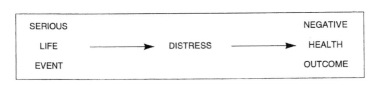

Figure 6.1 Life events and health outcomes

There are a number of factors that explain why one person copes better with a serious life event than another. Personality characteristics are one such factor. Another, which is the concern of this chapter, is the degree of social support available. For example, in Mrs McDonald's case the existence of social support may in various ways help relieve her distress about the death of her husband. Furthermore, her distress may not have a negative health outcome if there is a support network to help her through the period of grief and mourning. This is illustrated in Figure 6.2, which shows the 'stress-buffering' effect of social support. At the two ends of a spectrum, Mrs McDonald may have virtually no support or she may have a good supportive network comprising a range of relatives, neighbours and friends.

A number of studies give credence to the buffering role of social support (Gottlieb, 1983; Stewart, 1993; Cooper *et al.*, 1999). There is also evidence that social support has a positive direct effect on health (Gottlieb, 1983; Stewart, 1993), in that it fosters good health and good morale by fulfilling basic social needs. Thus, if Mrs McDonald has had a good supportive network around her for many years she will be in a healthier state and in better shape to cope with the distress of the bereavement than would otherwise be the case. As Litwin (1995, p. 156) states 'As is widely established in

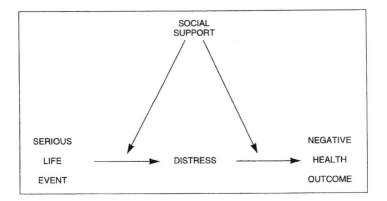

Figure 6.2 The stress-buffering effects of social support

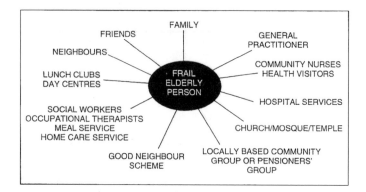

Figure 6.3 Circle of support for a frail older person

the literature, the informal social network can serve as an effective means of mitigating stress in a range of situations'. Halpern also concludes that 'it is generally accepted that intimate, confiding relationships act as a 'buffer' to protect individuals from the adversities of life' (2005, p. 76). Practitioners are frequently assisting people with life crises and life transitions so this area of social support is an important area to understand and appreciate.

Social support can of course come from different sources – both informal and formal. Family, friends and neighbours are the main source of most people's support but an older person may also obtain support from a range of other sources, for example good neighbour schemes, day centres, voluntary organisations, workers from the health or social services or the local mosque, temple or church. It is possible to represent these sources of support as a circle around the person, as shown in Figure 6.3. Some literature refers to these social resources and connections as 'social capital' (Field, 2003) and we will return to this shortly.

A key issue for health and social care workers is assessing the available support and intervening in a way that maximises such support for vulnerable people. One way in which social support can be looked at is in terms of 'networks'. Network analysis provides a clear way of understanding these connections and understanding social capital. This will also be examined in more detail later in the chapter but Figure 6.3 provides a starting point.

Social capital

Mention was made earlier of the idea of 'social capital', a concept which is increasingly referred to in the literature. It has particularly been popularised by David Putnam and some key ideas are outlined in Box 6.1.

Box 6.1 **Bowling Alone *with David Putnam***

David Putnam is a dominating author and voice on the topic of social capital. He defines social capital as 'connections among individuals – social networks and the norms of reciprocity and trustworthiness that arise from them' (2000, p. 19). He has popularised the concept, notably with his book, *Bowling Alone* (2000). The book depicts people disengaged from public life and disconnected from each other. He regards disengagement and disconnectedness as negative aspects of society that need redressing. The image is one of people in bowling lanes playing on their own and this image symbolised and popularised his notion that social capital was collapsing in the United States.

The book *Bowling Alone* outlines the trend towards civic disengagement in the United States and Putnam provides much data on the decline of connections in the workplace, informal social connections and of political, civic, and religious participation. There are some exceptions to this but Putnam argues that these do not outweigh the many ways in which Americans were less connected to their communities in the last third of the twentieth century than the previous two-thirds.

Putnam does not believe that the changing family structures or the growth of the welfare state have caused this decline. Among the factors which have contributed are pressures of time and money; suburbanisation, commuting and urban sprawl; the impact of electronic entertainment, especially television; and generational change – which has replaced an involved civic generation with less involved children and grandchildren.

Putnam draws out the links between social capital and aspects such as child development, crime, economic prosperity, health, and better government. For example, he writes on health, 'The more integrated we are with our community, the less likely we are to experience colds, heart attacks, strokes, cancer, depression, and premature death of all sorts' (2000, p. 326).

I have some hesitancy about using the language of 'social capital'. The notion of an investment which produces a return does not for me capture the sense of love, obligation and duty which so often is a part of human relationships. However, it has become the language that is used in much social science and social policy literature so it cannot be ignored. Clearly, government policy can affect social capital. It is sometimes said that the housing redevelopments of the 1950s often improved the housing conditions but did much to damage the social capital of people. In some places, these policies involved pulling down housing in inner city communities and dispersing people to new, outlying estates. Another example relates to the closure of long-stay hospitals. If these are poorly organised, they can damage and destroy the social capital of residents built up over many years. A third example would suggest that the social capital of people who are moved into institutions can be seriously affected by the change.

Strategies for partnership

One of the most useful attributes among community health and social care workers is the ability to identify, work with and enlarge service users' networks of support. Put another way, this is to actively work with an individual's social capital. Collins and Pancoast (1976) in their book on neighbourhood-based forms of informal support argued that natural helping networks were of great potential use in social welfare. Here the focus was on mutual aid, linking up with and making use of 'central figures' or 'natural neighbours'.

Biegel *et al.* (1984) developed this in relation to network approaches to working with older people. Froland *et al.* (1981) looked at strategies that agencies might adopt in order to maximise partnership with the informal sector. As noted in Chapter 2, there were others, such as Bayley (1973) and Bulmer (1987), who stressed the need for interweaving and partnership in their writing. Froland *et al.* (1981) suggested five strategies for welfare agencies that are still very relevant when considering care in the community.

Personal networks strategy

Once the details of a network are known, there may be different ways in which it can be modified to suit the user. Members of the network may hold meetings in order better to coordinate their activities. Sometimes it is possible to improve the functioning of the network. At other times it may be better to try to create new networks. If a worker is trying to help someone join a network, one of the following strategies may help.

Volunteer linking

There is a long tradition of voluntary welfare work. An example here is the Buddy Service, which provides friendship and support for people with HIV/AIDS. This was started by the Terence Higgins Trust in London but similar schemes have been set up throughout the United Kingdom. A Buddy is a volunteer who commits him or herself to befriending someone with HIV/AIDS and sees them perhaps two or three times a week. Training is given and each Buddy receives advice on befriending, listening and practical tasks.

Mutual aid networks

There is a vast number of self-help organisations and groups. This type of help can be very powerful because all of the members have had similar experiences. One of the oldest and best known is Alcoholics Anonymous. More recently, self-advocacy groups have been set up for people with learning difficulties. The internet has added another dimension to this with many people obtaining support and help through their computer.

Neighbourhood helper strategy

In any area there are usually a number of local people who take on a neighbourly helping role. This strategy involves the agency finding out who these people are and working with them. There may be occasions when they need support, but there may also be occasions when they can generate support and help for a vulnerable person through their local contacts and by virtue of their local leadership.

Community empowerment strategy

This is similar to mutual aid but usually involves a worker helping groups and communities to organise mutual aid, self-help and local empowerment. Because it involves collective organisation it is especially important as a strategy against oppressive structures and policies.

Often these strategies can be beneficially combined. The above categorisation into five strategies remains useful for looking at the different ways in which the formal sector can relate to the informal sector. They can all have a beneficial impact on an individual's social capital. There is a great deal of altruism within the community, and health and social care workers need to work with this and encourage it (Titmus, 1973) while endeavouring not to exploit people. Reflect on these strategies in relation to the case study in Box 6.2.

Box 6.2   Case study – application of partnership strategies

Peter has learning difficulties and has been in a long-stay hospital for 15 years. He is being moved with two other people to a small group home 12 miles from the hospital. When Peter is discharged from hospital, his network is likely to be dramatically changed. People who spend many years in hospital build up a network associated with the institution. In Peter's case that network will be fractured, prompting two important questions:

- Will anyone help him to keep in touch with the old network if he wishes to?
- Will he be able to build a new network up in his new situation?

In the interest of good care management practice, the maintenance of Peter's network will need to be actively thought about, supported and created. A number of the partnership strategies described above may be relevant. He may need help with keeping in touch with people who have been important to him (personal network strategy). Within his new community, linking him to a citizen advocacy scheme may be one way of helping him to build a network in his new situation (volunteer linking). Citizen advocacy is sometimes described as 'lending people networks'. This means linking someone to Peter as an advocate. Subsequently the members of the advocate's network will get to know Peter and in this way a network is 'lent'. There may be a self-advocacy group that Peter can join (mutual-aid networks). A knowledge of the new area in which Peter will be living may identify some local people who might provide a link for Peter into the new area (neighbourhood helper strategy). A worker may help Peter and others to play an active role in their new area (community empowerment).

Transitions and community care

The movement of Peter from a long-stay hospital into a small group home represented a major 'transition' in his life. Likewise with the earlier example of Mrs McDonald, the death of her husband represented a similar significant transition. All of us pass through these transitions in our lives – they happen, for example, when a loved one dies; when we have a significant change of job or at retirement; and when close relationships take a major change through perhaps a separation or a divorce. We all have experience of the stress, upset and pain. For a service user it is likely that a movement into residential care will represent a major transition. People vary and it may be that the first time a 'care worker' is needed in someone's home represents a big transition – signifying the loss of being able to look after themselves.

There are some models to help us understand transitions. Probably the best known is the 'stages model' associated with death and loss. It was suggested that dying people go through five stages of denial, anger, bargaining, depression and acceptance (Kubler-Ross, 1969). This model has been influential for practitioners and has been extended to grieving and loss more generally as well as modified in a number of ways (Thompson, 2002). While some can find this helpful others may point to the variety of human experience and the way in which both individuals and cultures vary in how they respond to situations.

Box 6.3   *Thinking about transitions*

Think of a person you know (or it could be yourself) who has been through a transition and it has continued to be felt as a bad and negative experience. Then try to think of someone who has been through a transition who has come through it with at least some positive feelings and aspects to it. Can you identify any factors that contributed to the transition remaining negative or factors that have contributed towards some positive aspects.

Community care practitioners are involved a lot with people going through transitions. If they can understand the processes better and then with their knowledge, skills and personality help people come through them more positively then this is an important element of practice. Mention was made above of the 'stages model' in relation to loss. This model has been very dominant and influential. Since the early 1990s, there have been challenges to this approach. Other models have developed (Thompson, 2002; Firth *et al.*, 2005). One model is the 'dual process' model (Stroebe and Schut, 1999) that identified two dimensions of experiencing loss:

- Loss orientation with a focus on the past. The focus here is on helping people face their grief and sense of loss.
- Restoration orientation with a focus on the present and the future. Here, the focus is on avoidance and doing practical things. It does involve keeping ties alive to the deceased and ties to the deceased are encouraged.

Both orientations are seen as being needed for adjustment to loss and people move between the two. To describe this movement between the two dimensions the term 'oscillation' is used. Thus within this model people suffering loss move between these two orientations, sometimes confronting and sometimes avoiding these dimensions of loss. Quinn writes, 'This model was welcomed by palliative care practitioners as offering a new approach, one which is matched by their observations in practice' (2005., p. 3).

People find different ways of coping at different times and the 'dual process' model readily allows for this. There may not be an end 'stage'. Silverman writes, 'Coping with the death of someone close to us may be a process that continues in different ways for the remainder of our lives' (2005, p. 30). Silverman also stresses how different writers have documented the importance of social support in facilitating effective coping. Thus one key element to the process of coping with a significant transition is the existence and the performance of an individual's support network and we will turn to this next.

What is meant by network?

Earlier in this chapter the concept of social capital was introduced. Halpern (2005, p. 10) argues that social capital is 'composed of a network, a cluster of norms, values and expectations shared by group members, and sanctions (punishments and rewards) that help to maintain both the norms and the network'. This emphasis on network within social capital is shared by Phillipson *et al.* (2004, p. 3) who write, 'Social capital can be roughly understood in terms of the social resources and connections that an individual has at his or her disposal and network analysis provides an elegant and visual way of understanding these resources and connections'. This section focuses on what a 'network' is and what network analysis is.

The word 'network' is often used interchangeably with 'support' but it also has a more precise definition, drawing from the methodology of network analysis in the social sciences. Network analysis is a research strategy and a sophisticated way of analysing relationships. It is generally considered to have its origins in social anthropology (e.g., Barnes, 1954; Bott, 1957). For those living at home and experiencing increased incapacity, there are important questions about what sort of network they have, how it changes and whether it can cope with increasing pressure and demand. Some of the ideas of network analysis can be helpful for practitioners in relation both to the analysis of situations and to practice. Many people stay in the community because their networks are sufficiently strong to cope with the demands. It is often because networks can no longer cope that admission to residential, nursing home or hospital care is required. It is also worth bearing in mind that not all network links are supportive. As a way of understanding what networks are and making them more real for yourself, carry out the exercise in Box 6.4.

Networks can be very different. In the centre of the network in Figure 6.4 is the recently bereaved Mrs McDonald who was introduced at the beginning of the chapter. She is frail, partially sighted and has a number of medical problems. She has a network size of four: her son, who lives over one hundred miles away and visits about every three months, or more often in a crisis; a daily home help; an Age Concern 'good neighbour';

Box 6.4 Drawing up a network

On a large sheet of paper draw a circle with yourself in the middle. Around yourself write the names of those with whom you have a relationship and to whom you could turn for help and support. Those who are closest to you should be placed nearest the centre. Do this before you read on.

- How many people have you put in your personal network? This is called the network *size*.
- How is your network made up in relation to divisions such as friends, neighbours and colleagues? This is called the network *composition*.
- How well do the people in your network know each other? This is called the network *density*. (If they know each other well it is a high-density network. If they do not know each other well it is a low-density network.)

---

and a next-door neighbour. They all know each other well so there is a high density. This means that when a difficulty arises they are quickly in touch with each other and cooperate to provide appropriate help or support.

Contrast this network with the network diagram in Figure 6.5. This network has the same composition but none of the people know each other (there is a low density) and they do not communicate with each other. (In reality this is unlikely but it illustrates the contrast with Figure 6.4.) It is much harder to see how Mrs McDonald could survive in the community with so little cooperation between those who support her. The members of

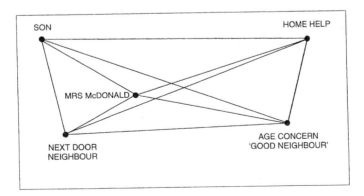

Figure 6.4 A high-density network

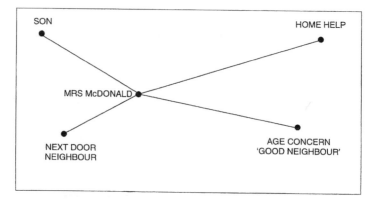

Figure 6.5 A low-density network

the network would not cover the gaps or back each other up when there were problems.

In a situation such as this, it might be helpful to organise a network meeting. With the user's permission the central members of the network are drawn together for a discussion. This meeting can help clarify who is doing what; identify any weak parts of the network and help the network members to link up and get to know each other. People who have never met or coordinated their efforts may begin to do so. In this way, an effective inter-weaving of formal and informal care can be achieved. Some key questions to pose in relation to practice are as follows:

- Is there a good reason for convening the meeting?
- Has the practitioner prepared well for the meeting and does he or she know the reasons for it?
- Has the user been fully involved in the discussions about the meeting and who is invited? The user normally attends unless there is a good reason why this should not be the case.
- Is the meeting likely to be constructive? If one of the network members is, for example, very negative for whatever reason, it may not be helpful to have the meeting.

A 'review' of a care package may invite the range of people involved and serve the purpose of a network meeting without being called such. I have attended such a 'review' where a neighbour said 'the network is working well'. Where a care manager draws up a care plan outlining everyone's contribution then (with permissions) telephone numbers and addresses can be a part of this, thus encouraging and facilitating the process. Everyone then receives a copy of the care plan and can more easily link up with each other if they need to.

The nature of the network

This section provides ideas on how to work out the details of networks as a practitioner. The following exercise requires you to choose someone who is already being worked with, preferably a frail, older person. The idea is to try to find out about his or her network. This is often done by generating names through a series of questions (Fischer, 1982). Write down who helps the person in question, if anyone, with practical tasks such as:

- Cleaning the house
- Cooking
- Washing dishes
- Laundry
- Gardening
- Household repairs
- Household decorations
- Shopping
- Pension collection
- Transportation

List who helps, if anyone, with personal care tasks such as:

- Bathing
- Washing
- Dressing
- Going to the toilet
- Getting into bed
- Feeding
- Shaving/hair combing
- Cutting toenails
- Negotiating steps/stairs
- Getting around the house
- Getting out of doors

Ask the person in question the following questions on

- Who can you confide in about problems?
- Who would you call real friends?
- Who depends on your friendship?
- Who do you keep in touch with over the telephone?

This list of questions (or some variation of it) is a quick way of obtaining an idea of the people in someone's network. It takes into account both formal and informal sources of support. The checklist is particularly applicable to frail older people. For other people it may well have to be modified. Having drawn up the list, show it to the person and ask them if there is anyone not on the list who gives help and support.

Adding up the list gives the *size* of the person's network. The *composition* is determined by whether the people on it are from the formal sector (social worker, GP, community nurse) or the informal sector (friends, neighbours). The *density* of the network depends on the extent to which those in the network know each other. In practical terms, this can be determined by listing the network members along the top and down the side of a sheet of paper. 'Does X know Y?' is asked in relation to each possible relationship (Fischer, 1982).

It needs to be said that examining someone's personal network is just one way of measuring support, and the method of measuring the network described above is only one way of doing this. However the practice of obtaining names from the person and asking about those names is common.

Returning to the exercise, the size, composition and an idea of the density of the person's network have now been established. Taking each member of the network individually, is there anything else it would be interesting to know about them? It could be important to ask the person concerned the following questions:

- How often do you see them? (Frequency)
- How long have you known them? (Duration)
- How far away do they live? (Proximity)
- How close do they feel to the person? (Closeness)
- How prominent or important is the person in the network? (Prominence) (Sharkey, 1989)

The answers to these questions need to be considered as a whole. In some cases, for example, the person concerned may not get on very well with a relative who lives nearby and visits often, but feels close to and able to discuss things with a relative who lives some distance away but keeps in touch by phone.

There is a range of other questions that could be asked to help fill out the picture of the person's network. Once you have the network map (it is a good idea to draw it as a diagram) you and the person concerned might be able to identify aspects that might helpfully be changed.

Different types of network

It will have become clear that practitioners need to go beyond simply saying that they acknowledge the value of informal care and will work with it. They need knowledge of how it works, how it varies and the implications of that variation for practice. They need to know how to assess it and how to link their intervention or care packages most effectively to it.

Wenger's (1994) work on the types of network that exist is helpful in developing this knowledge and skill. She argues that different patterns of informal support exist in the community and that different types of neighbourhood produce different types of network and patterns of help-seeking behaviour. Certain aspects of help or support networks have been identified as crucial (Wenger and Day, 1995):

- How close the network members live to one another.
- How many members know each other.
- Which informal sources are turned to for help.

In her study of older people in North Wales, Wenger (1984) found that support networks had an average of five to seven members, although the range was from two to 22. She developed a measurement instrument for practitioner identification of network type and tested the usefulness of this as a practice tool. Five types of support network were identified on the basis of the following factors:

- Local availability of close kin.
- Level of involvement of family, friends and neighbours.
- Level of interaction with the community and voluntary groups.

The networks are named according to the nature of the older person's relationship to the network. The first three types are based on the presence of local kin, the other two reflect their absence:

- Family dependent.
- Local integrated.
- Local self-contained.
- Wider community focused.
- Private restricted.

Wenger argues that different types of network make different demands on the statutory services. For example the level of domiciliary care required differs according to network type. Network types themselves change over time. At different times communities have differing proportions of network types, with likely implications for the services provided. Only some networks can adapt to support highly dependent older people in need of long-term care.

When older people have problems or needs, how they are responded to and how they are met depends on the type of network available. Wenger discusses this in relation to problems resulting from impaired mobility, illness, hospital discharge, the impact of widowhood, isolation and loneliness, dementia/mental illness. She also indicates how different network types are likely to perceive and use services such as home care, meals, good neighbour schemes, community nursing, day care, respite care and residential care (Wenger and Day, 1995).

The key message from Wenger's work is that practitioners need to work to support or complement the existing networks. Workers should not simply consider the person concerned, their problems and the available services when designing a care package. They should also take full account of the support network, and knowledge of the network type can assist with the planning of services. In an evaluative study, the use of network assessments related to the typology were shown to be much appreciated and valued by two social work teams in South Wales (Wenger and Tucker, 2002).

Other attempts have been made to develop network typologies. For example, Litwin has related the different network types available to older people in Israel to the use of health services (Litwin, 1997), health status (Litwin, 1998) and the use of both formal and informal help (Litwin, 1999).

Working with networks in community care practice

It is often because the informal network is under great strain that a situation is brought to the attention of the formal services. The services need to have some sense of how the network is working before a decision is made on the way forward. Litwin (1995) outlines four models of network intervention, although he acknowledges that in practice they overlap and are not distinct. These are:

- Network therapy: this draws on the perspectives of family therapy.
- Network mediation: this might involve, for example, expanding networks and increasing the connections between them.
- Network construction: this involves building a network where none or only a very small one exists.
- Network reinforcement: here a network under strain receives support or back-up from the paid services. This is similar to the notion employed by some writers and practitioners of interweaving informal and formal care.

There is some tradition of working with networks rather than just individuals, and a history of practice in different countries to draw on (Trimble and Kliman, 1995). Pioneers of this approach in the United States include Attneave (1969), Rueveni (1979) and Speck (Speck and Attneave, 1973). In a brief review of literature, Kawachi and Berkman (2001, p. 464) note some successes in interventions with support groups, one-to-one support interventions and interventions to enhance natural networks.

Mention has been made of changing the density of a network by, for example, convening a meeting or a series of meetings of those involved within the network. Networks can be very fragile and the meetings may reveal that there is a need for the support and maintenance of informal carers. Perhaps those at the meetings will help to provide this, or alternatives may be explored. Sometimes one member of a network can feel overloaded and there is a need to try to reduce the pressure. It may become clear that the network is too small. The size of a network might be increased by recruiting a volunteer or a good neighbour. Advocates for people with learning disabilities or people who are mentally distressed often add to the size of networks through mutual involvement in ordinary leisure activities.

Heron (1998) applies similar ideas in her study of carers. She describes the valuable role that support groups can play for carers and suggests that carers may benefit from an improvement of their social networks. She suggests two stages for the latter – first the mapping of the existing network (similar to the method described above) and then a discussion of options for developing the network using new and existing contacts.

Network therapy is one of the approaches used for treating people who abuse alcohol and drugs (Galanter, 1999). Family members and friends are involved in the treatment so that they can provide support and promote a change of attitude. One function of Alcoholics Anonymous is to provide a support network of people who are committed to giving up alcohol. Replacing a 'drinking network' with a network of people who are determined to stop drinking can be a crucial step along the road to recovery.

Social networks shape high-risk behaviour and thus the spread of HIV. Friedman's (1999) study shows that social networks are of vital importance in understanding and fighting HIV/AIDS. Understanding networks is thus important in this and other areas of preventive healthcare.

The concepts of networks and social capital are useful in analysing the situation of refugees and refugee organisations (Griffiths *et al.*, 2005). People who migrate leave behind networks and social capital. In their new situation, they need networks and social capital to survive. Policies of dispersal need to be considered in the light of this.

Practice in community care needs to be based on a careful analysis of the current support available from both the formal and the informal sector in order to achieve a sensible and sensitive interweaving of care. Herein lie some of the real skills of care management as the process is not cold and technocratic but rather demands considerable assessment and intervention skills. There will be some situations where the current network is very limited and fragile and a considerable input of formal services will be needed. However, there will be other situations where the activities of the current network can simply be modified to meet needs. Sometimes, for example, the provision of appropriate guidance, training or reassurance by district nurses to carers may be all that is required. Intervention by practitioners will vary according to the assessment but could be directed at:

- Strengthening the current support system.
- Creating a new support system.
- Training users in the skills necessary to help them strengthen their own support system.

Practice issues

This chapter has covered a number of terms such as community, social support, social capital and networks. There are both overlaps between these terms and some differences. Some familiarity with them is important for practitioners because they all have relevance to the situations dealt with by health and social care practitioners and can help with reflections on appropriate practice.

In *Integrating Social Support in Nursing*, Stewart (1993) details the links between social support, social networks and health. She applies social support to the four stages of decision-making in nursing – assessment, planning, intervention and evaluation. Stewart outlines a nursing approach based on social support where users and carers are viewed as partners and allies. She stresses a collaborative approach that goes beyond rhetoric to the need for a detailed analysis of the support network:

> 'If you say your practice includes assessment of the social network prior to discharge of a patient, state exactly what you will assess: size? frequency of contact? degree of conflict? density? satisfaction? perceived available support? If you determine a social support deficit or disfunction, be specific about its indicators and, if appropriate, your planned intervention.' (Tilden in Stewart, 1993, p. 204)

Stewart draws on a large body of literature to show the importance of support networks for health outcomes and makes a powerful argument in favour of nurses knowing about and working constructively with support networks. The need for knowledge about and skills in networking applies to all workers in the broad area of health promotion (Trevillion, 1999).

A call for partnership can also be found in the influential Griffiths Report on community care: 'Families, friends, neighbours and other local people provide the majority of care in response to needs which they are uniquely well placed to identify and respond to. This will continue to be the primary means by which people are enabled to live normal lives in community settings' (Griffiths, 1988, p. 5). The report took this as its starting point, and recommended that publicly provided services should support and where possible strengthen these networks of carers (ibid., p 5).

Historically, nursing and social work seem to have blown hot and cold at different times over their relations with communities/local networks. There is almost a cyclical pattern to this. Earlier chapters have stressed how during the 1990s, due to the legislative changes and the impact of internal markets, pressure was put on practitioners to undertake individual work, with less attention to community/network factors. The emphasis during the 1990s of 'targeting those in greatest need' contributed to some loss of emphasis on support networks. However, this was balanced by government rhetoric on and acknowledgement of the role played in community care by informal carers (DoH, 1989a). Thus practitioners have again found themselves in an ambivalent situation, with competing pressures and tensions.

This chapter has also discussed the links between life events, social support and health outcomes. Much of the work of community care practitioners concerns issues of loss, suffering and transition. Service users may well have their own explanations and/or religious understandings of major life transitions such as death and loss and it is important for practitioners to appreciate these and be sensitive to them. In helping people in these situations or in helping carers, practitioners can draw on what is known about loss and transitions. The emphasis of this chapter has been on the importance of support and networks at these times. Networks are an important aspect of coping with life crises, coping with deteriorating health and continuing to live in the community. Thus key tasks for care managers are to:

- assess the users' current support networks, and
- take action to ensure that the support networks continue, with appropriate assistance.

Practitioners might make use of this chapter by working with service users to assess their networks so that any agreed intervention or way forward can be informed by this background knowledge. It is an appropriate approach for a wide range of service users (Whittaker and Garbarino, 1983). Hill (2002) has described in detail how he built teaching on it into basic social work training.

Network analysis is helpful for the care manager in terms of analysing the current network and assisting with sorting out how the successful interweaving of formal and informal care can take place. It is acknowledged that it may be difficult if there is pressure for a quick assessment from a practitioner on the purchasing side of the purchaser/provider divide. However, assessments are not static and later involvement and/or later 'reviews' may allow more time for this. Domiciliary care package 'reviews' offer an opportunity to check how the whole support network is operating and that the different members of it are able to contact each other if necessary.

It is useful for practitioners to reflect on the following (Wenger, 1994):

- People with different types of network are likely to make different degrees and types of demand on statutory services.
- Knowledge and understanding of the various types of support network can be a useful tool for community care practitioners at the level of the individual and the team.

The telephone has been enormously beneficial in respect of maintaining networks and enabling people to obtain support when needed. Increasing numbers of people are keeping in touch through the internet and electronic mail. It seems likely that we will see more communication through new technology as a way of developing networks and obtaining support.

Further reading

Two books which give an overview of the background to the concept of social capital and the debates around it are:

Field, J. (2003) *Social Capital* (London: Routledge).
Halpern, D. (2005) *Social Capital* (Cambridge: Polity Press).

Two books that offer helpful collections of chapters for practitioners on aspects of transition, loss and grief are:

Thompson, N. (ed.) (2002) *Loss and Grief* (London: Palgrave).
Firth, P., G. Luff and D. Oliviere (eds) (2005) *Loss, Change and Bereavement in Palliative Care* (London: Open University Press).

Phillipson, C., G. Allan and D. Morgan (2004) *Social Networks and Social Exclusion* (Aldershot: Ashgate). This book gives an overview of debates on the contributions of social networks to social capital and social exclusion.

World Wide Web site

The chapter mentioned sources of support through the internet. There are many sources available. One example would be an on-line grief support network at www.griefnet.org. This site hosts over forty different support groups with members throughout the world.

CHAPTER 7

User Empowerment and Community Care

Chapter summary

This chapter:

- Discusses some key influences on empowerment in community care including the independent living movement and direct payments; the social model of disability; normalisation, ordinary living and person-centred planning; the self-help and user movement; and community development.
- Outlines two models of empowerment and describes a 'ladder of empowerment'.
- Situates community care in a wider context and considers debates on social exclusion and regeneration.

Introduction

Previous chapters have referred to the recognition of user empowerment in the community care changes of the 1990s. It has been pointed out (for example, in Chapter 4) that this has often conflicted with other objectives, including the rationing of services and the provision of services within tight budgets. This chapter explores the welcome emphasis on empowerment, but this needs to be considered in the wider context that includes the often complex and varied expectations that practitioners have to meet. User involvement can be applied to all situations of community care in some way. As an illustration, Box 7.1 mentions a study where it is applied to people who are seriously ill.

Box 7.1   *User empowerment and seriously ill people*

Issues of user empowerment apply across the whole range of situations covered by community care. A study called *Too Ill To Talk* (Small and Rhodes, 2000)

---

assessed the concept of user involvement in services for people who suffer from multiple sclerosis, motor neurone disease and cystic fibrosis. Some issues that I drew from it were:

- User-involvement is important across the whole range of services dealing with living and dying.
- The importance of retaining some control over the process of dying and death. There may be issues about choice of place of death. Euthanasia is not legally acceptable in United Kingdom but some influence on the process of dying may be important to the patient.
- The research study had the notion of people leaving a legacy by influencing services for others after they had died.
- The importance of recognising that some people living with a serious illness may have more pressing concerns and may actively choose not to take part in user involvement.

One of the three fundamental aims of *Caring for People*, was to 'give people a greater individual say in how they live their lives and the services they need to help them to do so' (DoH, 1989a, p. 4). Later practice guidance from the Department of Health further emphasised involving service users and increasing their choices. The language of empowerment is employed to promote this objective:

'The rationale for this reorganisation is the empowerment of users and carers. Instead of users and carers being subordinate to the wishes of service providers, the roles will be progressively adjusted. In this way, users and carers will be enabled to exercise the same power as consumers of other services. This redressing of the balance of power is the best guarantee of a continuing improvement in the quality of service.' (DoH, 1991a, p. 9)

The aspects of user empowerment that were built into the community care changes of the early 1990s can be summarised as follows:

- Users were to receive better information about services and procedures.
- Each social service authority was required to set up a complaints procedure for users.
- There was to be consultation with users in relation to community care plans.
- Assessment of individuals was to be guided by the needs of the user.

Although the changes were useful in themselves in practice they only had a limited impact on empowerment. The empowerment envisaged was mainly strengthening the individual's right to (1) complain, (2) better information and (3) needs-led assessment. The scope for collective organisation was limited to participation in community care plans and whatever could be made of the general rhetoric of user empowerment.

It is clear that there was only limited government encouragement of user empowerment. Since then a variety of other influences on community care have had a greater impact on real empowerment. Foremost among these are:

- The independent living movement and direct payments.
- The influence of the social model of disability.
- Ideas about normalisation, ordinary living, and person-centred planning.
- The continuing development of the user movement and self-help groups.
- The influence of community work ideas and practices.

There has been an interlinking of these influences so that they have all had an impact on each other in different ways. The first five sections of this chapter will outline each of these influences in turn. What follows however cannot show the complexity of this interlinking or the detail of the debates that have taken place. All of them have contributed to the development of good practice. It must be remembered that practitioners have also had to struggle with resource constraints, which frequently serve to limit empowerment.

Independent living movement and direct payments

In the United States during the 1960s, discrimination was identified as a major problem in relation to black people, women and disabled people. Disability thus became an issue of concern to the civil rights movement. The links between oppressed groups were made more explicit in the United States than in the United Kingdom. The movement of disabled people in the United States has sometimes been called the Independent Living Movement and there have been examples of disabled people taking service provision into their own hands, for instance the first Center For Independent Living was set up in Berkeley, California, in 1972 (Crewe and Zola, 1983). Other centres were opened during the subsequent years. A central aim was to 'demedicalise' disability, that is, to put a stop to disability being treated as akin to sickness.

The movement has been slower to develop in the United Kingdom. It had its origins in people's attempts to leave residential care and live independently in the community. Examples of important initiatives are the Derbyshire Centre for Integrated Living, the Hampshire Centre for Independent Living and the West of England Centre for Inclusive Living. The Derbyshire Centre for Integrated Living was set up in the early 1980s. It was run and managed by disabled people for disabled people with a mission is to secure independent, integrated living opportunities for disabled people in order to promote their full participation in the mainstream of economic life in Derbyshire. Further details of its history and development can be found in Priestley (1999).

Box 7.2   Centres for independent living

The Prime Minister's Strategy Unit's report *Improving the Life Chances of Disabled People* (2005), reported that there were 22 fully constituted centres for independent living (CIL) and another 15 local disability organisations either providing a similar role or working towards becoming such a centre. For most CILS, their main activity and source of income is running support schemes to assist and enable disabled people to use direct payments.

According to Jenny Morris (1993), the philosophy of the independent living movement is based on the following assumptions: that all human life is of value; that anyone, whatever their impairment, is capable of making choices; that people who are disabled by society's reaction to physical, intellectual and sensory impairment and emotional distress have the right to assert control over their lives; and that disabled people have the right to participate fully in society (ibid., p. 21).

Independent disabled people (as in the independent living movement) argue that they are in charge of decision-making even if they do not do all the tasks themselves (for example, getting washed and dressed). The reversal of the power relationship is achieved by moving away from disabled people being controlled by personal assistance (however kind and well-meaning) towards control over the type and timing of the personal assistance they receive. That is, disabled people themselves decide which services they want (such as help with getting up, going to bed, eating) and when they want them. The physical inability to do certain tasks should not lead to loss of control and choice. What is important is the nature of the relationship with the person who is doing the tasks. This relates to who is in charge of what is done, how it is done and when it is done. Obviously there can be tensions between this philosophy and the way in which caring has been done in the past by many carers – both formal and informal. This potential and real conflict was brought out at the end of Chapter 2 and practitioners may experience conflicting pressures between the aspirations of disabled people and the concerns of carers.

The setting up by the UK government of the Independent Living Fund (ILF) in 1988 gave a boost to the independent living movement. Disabled people who could meet the assessment criteria were given a regular grant that enabled them to employ people to help them live independently. Hence, the fund gave disabled people control over their own care by enabling them to employ the carers of their choice and tell them what to do. This was very different from having to accept the dictates and organisation of the local home care and nursing service. Power shifted to the disabled person. In this way, the fund fed into the aims of the Independent Living Movement and provided a vision of how user-led and user-controlled care packages could be set up to meet the real needs of disabled people.

The closure of the ILF in its original form in 1993 provoked a great deal of anger among disabled people as it had provided them with greater control over their own lives as well as independence, and for many its removal meant a real reduction in possibilities for empowerment. During the early 1990s, there was a lot of pressure on the government by organisations of disabled people to legislate on direct payments and this pressure eventually bore fruit with the passing of the Community Care (Direct Payments) Act 1996.

Direct payments (DPs) is the system in the United Kingdom where individuals are given the money to chose and pay for their own social care rather than have directly provided services. Employing and directing personal assistants has always been central to the notion of direct payments. They are a means by which disabled people and older people can maintain control of their lives and there is a developing literature on what needs to be in place to enable it to work (Hasler and Stewart, 2004).

There have been concerns about the implementation of the policy. A report by the English Commission for Social Care Inspection (CSCI) in 2004 recorded the low take-up of direct payments and the great variability between authorities. The CSCI noted that since April 2003, English councils had been required to offer direct payments to anyone using community care services who could consent to the scheme. The report suggested that a combination of incompetence, lack of information, patronising attitudes and unhelpful paperwork had stalled the direct payments changes.

While there is a remarkable consensus on the merits (and contribution to empowerment) of independent living and direct payments, it is necessary to maintain some critical perspectives. Spandler notes how there are elements of various strands within DPs. She writes, 'The history of DPs has therefore comprised a complex confluence of new right, New Labour and welfare user movement ideologies and demands' (2004, p. 190). In an overview of the positives and the negatives of DPs, Spandler (2004) cautions that a number of factors need to be addressed in order to ensure DPs continue to be a progressive strategy. Such an individualistic approach could undercut collective notions of provision. Direct Payments might also lead to greater privatisation and there can be concern about the rights and conditions of workers under direct payments schemes (ibid.). Another writer has suggested that there may also be dangers of governments using this provision to cut back on other programmes and to increase pressure on families to look after their elderly relatives (Oldman, 2003). One study suggested that DPs might be a way of creating a more integrated and seamless service for people while at the same time contributing to the shift of funding responsibilities from health to social care (Glendinning *et al.*, 2000). Scourfield (2005) endorses the principles underlying DPs but raises questions about whether there will be an adequate supply of personal assistants and considers some of the concerns in relation to personal assistants around risk, training and regulation. This intriguing and important debate will go on – not least because the English government's Green Paper on adult social care (DoH, 2005b) clearly envisaged a much more central role for DPs within welfare provision in the future. This was confirmed in the subsequent White Paper (DoH, 2006).

Discussion about DPs has merged into discussion about 'individual budgets'. Take up of DPs was somewhat disappointing and it is acknowledged that some people and some groups do did not wish to have the burdens associated with them. Becoming an employer and taking on these responsibilities are very real barriers for many people. Both the Green Paper (DoH, 2005b) and the White Paper (DoH, 2006) discussed 'individual budgets' as a way forward that would reduce these barriers. The 'individual budget' would be held by the local authority on behalf of the service user. By this approach some resources are allocated to an individual based on an assessment of their individual need. Service users with individual budgets could ask councils to hold and administer payments for them. Service users can also buy council run services with their personal budgets, which they cannot do with DPs. Support is provided to help the person decide what they want and they can choose to receive support by the provision of services or by way of a cash payment. A number of pilot projects were to test out the way forward. In many situations practitioners would be less care managers but more navigators, facilitators or brokers.

The social model of disability

People involved in the independent living movement have often used the social model of disability as a theoretical perspective. The two influences on empowerment are intertwined. As one example, the Derbyshire Coalition for Inclusive Living says that its action programme is based on a social model of disability. What does this mean?

A model is a simplified version of how things operate and can help make sense of a complicated situation. Two models can be used to explain how disability is regarded by society. The first is the 'individual model', in which a disabled person is seen as having to adjust to society. (This model is sometimes called the medical model, the traditional model or the personal tragedy model.) Central aspects of this model are that disability is viewed as a 'tragic' situation; individuals have to adapt to their impairment; individuals have to adapt to fit into society; and disabled people may be seen as either objects of pity or heroes (Oliver and Sapey, 2006).

In contrast, under the 'social oppression model' society is expected to adjust to the disabled person. This model is advocated by a number of disabled persons' organisations and writers (e.g., Oliver 1990, 1996). From this perspective disabled people are seen primarily as an oppressed group, prevented from achieving their full potential by the structures of society and the language and belief systems which society develops about disabled people and their lives. Society 'disables' individuals both by creating environmental obstacles and by its attitude towards them. For example, disabled people have the same range of needs and feelings as other people but society restricts their access to public transport, entertainment and public places as well as education and employment. According to this approach, action should be taken to enable disabled people to play a full and equal part in all aspects of life.

These two models simplify complex situations but they nevertheless have fundamental implications for disabled people, their carers and the organisation of services provided for them. The model adopted will affect how practitioners behave and the way in which they practice. It is probable that most people have been heavily influenced by a portrayal of disability that conforms largely to the first model and is constantly reinforced by the media and some charities.

The social model does not stress the restrictions created by impairments, but rather the restrictions created by a society geared to able-bodied people. It shows how society denies disabled people the means to do what they are capable of doing. Hence, the problem is not the impaired individual but the disabling society. This model emphasises the need to identify the way in which the structures and institutions of society further disable people with disabilities so that these disabling structures can be challenged. The social model celebrates difference and has related in the past especially to people with a physical or a sensory impairment.

Proponents of the social model have been critical of those involved in the 'rehabilitation' services for medicalising the rehabilitation process

(Nocon and Baldwin, 1998). Health and social care workers in rehabilitation services have had to rethink their practices as a result of these criticisms. This also applies in respect of the influence of the ideas of normalisation.

Normalisation, ordinary living and person-centred planning

Normalisation has been especially influential in relation to services for people with learning difficulties, an area of provision in which the social model of disability has had only a limited impact (Stalker *et al.*, 1999). In the past people with learning difficulties were often shut away in large hospitals as a result of policies of physical exclusion and segregation. The ideas of 'normalisation' grew as a way of combating segregation and integrating people with learning difficulties back into society. Its origins were in Denmark in the late 1950s and the ideas influenced the provision of services in Denmark and Sweden in the 1960s. In the United States, during the 1970s and the 1980s, Wolf Wolfensberger (1972) proposed and then developed more elaborate ideas on normalisation, which he later referred to as 'social role valorisation'. This is his preferred description but the word 'normalisation' is still commonly used.

The aim of normalisation is simply to treat all people as equal citizens, with equal rights and equal access to valued social roles. The ideas of normalisation are applied to groups of people who have been regarded as of lesser value and suggest how to change that situation. Members of such groups are likely to be treated unfairly and unjustly, thus discrimination is one consequence of being devalued.

A vicious circle can be set up in which people who are seen and treated as being of lesser value come to believe it themselves. That is, when people hear negative views about themselves and experience negative behaviour, then over time they come to accept that view of themselves. Another word for this is 'internalisation'. Normalisation is one tool for identifying, analysing and breaking the circle that traps various groups of people into maintaining poor views of themselves and discourages their aspiration to be valued members of society. This can happen to people who are elderly, people who have a physical, sensory or learning disability and people with mental health problems. Thus the ideas of normalisation are relevant to all adult groups in the field of community care.

Normalisation principles have been a force for change in the United Kingdom, and in particular they have contributed to the 'ordinary life' movement. This movement is based on the conviction that people with severe learning difficulties should live ordinary lives. John O'Brien (King's Fund Centre, 1991) has described the implications of normalisation in relation to what services should try to achieve or accomplish for users. He has identified five major service accomplishments that are a practical application of the 'ordinary life' values for people with learning difficulties (ibid., p. 45):

- Community presence: the right to live and spend their time in the community rather than in residential, day or leisure facilities that segregate them from other members of society.
- Competence: in order for a full and rewarding life to be lived in the local community, many will require help with learning new skills and gaining access to a wider range of activities.
- Choice: a high-quality service will give priority to enhancing the choices available to people and generally protecting their human rights.
- Respect: services can play an important role in helping people to enjoy the same status as other valued members of society.
- Relationships: help and encouragement are needed to enable people with learning difficulties to mix with other non-disabled people in their daily lives.

These have been powerful and radical principles when applied to much of the provision which has been available for people with learning difficulties. Since the 1970s, people with learning difficulties have progressed towards living ordinary lives in a whole variety of areas, such as education, housing, employment and leisure. To use a more recent term, normalisation has acted as a powerful tool against social exclusion.

According to some interpretations of normalisation the devalued group is expected to adopt the culture and lifestyle of the dominant group (this process is sometimes called assimilation). However, while oppressed groups want to be valued as human beings, they might not wish to follow an approach that sees assimilation as the only goal or assumes that disadvantaged groups should aspire to society's norms (Szivos, 1992, p. 128).

In summary then, whereas the social model acknowledges and celebrates difference, normalisation has often appeared to emphasise assimilation. Szivos suggests that at a practical level, health and social care workers might ask themselves whether their way of working improves 'the self-concept of [the] client by acknowledging his or her right to feel positively about being different?' (ibid.)

Various White Papers and strategies have been published to further inform and guide practice. In England, *Valuing People* (DoH, 2001b), was published. *The Same as You* (Scottish Executive, 1999b) was published in Scotland and *Fulfilling the Promises* (Learning Disabilities Advisory Group, 2000) was produced in Wales. In many policy documents, the previous language of normalisation, social role valorisation and ordinary living has often been replaced by the language of 'person-centred approaches' – approaches that are intended to enable people with learning disabilities as much choice and control as possible over their lives. Mansell and Beadle-Brown write, 'Person-centred planning is an approach to organising assistance to people with intellectual disabilities. Developed over nearly 30 years in the United States, it has recently assumed particular importance in the United Kingdom because it forms a central component of the 2001 White Paper *Valuing People*' (2004).

The two sets of guidance associated with the English White Paper both had 'person centred' within their titles (DoH, 2002a, 2002b). In this guidance, the Department of Health defines person centred planning as, 'a process for continual listening, focusing on what is important to someone now and in the future, and acting upon this in alliance with family and friends' (2002b, p. 12). The guidance acknowledges different planning styles and planning tools and that these can be used for the process. It stresses that there are five key features that help to distinguish it from other forms of planning and assessment. These are outlined in Box 7.3.

Box 7.3 Five key features of person-centred planning

The following five features are said to distinguish person-centred planning from other forms of planning:

- 'The person is at the centre.
- Family members and friends are full partners.
- Person-centred planning reflects the person's capacities, what is important to a person (now and for their future) and specifies the support they may require to make a valued contribution to their community.
- Person-centred planning builds a shared commitment to action that will uphold the person's rights.
- Person-centred planning leads to continual listening, learning and action, and helps the person get what they want out of life'.

(DoH, 2002b, pp. 13–14)

This is a developing area of policy and practice with ongoing debate as to whether it will deliver what it intends (Mansell and Beadle-Brown, 2004). The Department of Health guidance (DoH, 2002b) is a source of further information and Ritchie *et al.* (2003) have produced a helpful practical guide for would-be implementers of person centred planning. The language of 'person-centred' and 'person-centred planning' is also used in relation to other users of community care service users (DoH, 2001c).

The growth of self-help groups, user groups and movements

There is a long history of self-help and self-organisation among users of community care services. The British Deaf Association was formed in 1890 and the National League of the Blind was set up as a trade union in 1899. This rich history can be explored in works such as 'Disability Politics' (Campbell and Oliver, 1996). A number of writers describe this history in terms of the development of a social movement (Beresford, 1997; Campbell and Oliver, 1996; Priestley, 1999). Some disabled people see it as a liberation movement (Oliver, 1996). The disability movement has been greatly influenced by the social model of disability and the idea of independent living, and the two have become inextricably bound together.

While the history of self-organisation goes back a long way (Campbell and Oliver, 1996), there has been considerable growth of disabled people's and service users' groups since the 1970s (Beresford, 1997). The growth and development of the independent living movement was discussed earlier in the chapter. There are numerous lessons to be learnt from the growth of self-help and user groups. Organisations have usually followed the principles and values of community development by emphasising collective organisation and self-organisation. The concept of community has been based on a 'community of interest' rather than a geographical area, but it nonetheless utilises the principles of community development. Self-advocacy, for example, happens when people speak and act on their own behalf and take a more active role in their own community (Williams and Shoultz, 1982). The emergence of self-advocacy groups such as People First has been a significant development in recent decades.

People First encourages people with learning difficulties to take control of their own lives. It began in North America and was started in the United Kingdom in the mid-1980s. The organisation has local groups and a national office that supports the development of self-advocacy. Many self-advocacy groups are associated with it. The groups are made up of people with learning difficulties and are often based in training centres, hostels and special schools. The growth of these groups has been influenced by the ideas surrounding normalisation and social role valorisation mentioned previously (Brandon, 1995).

There are now a number of other national umbrella organisations for user groups and self-help groups. The British Council of Organisations of Disabled People is one example of this. User organisations played an important part in bringing about the direct payments legislation and the anti-discrimination legislation (Priestley, 1999). Carers UK is an umbrella organisation for carers' groups and was an active lobbyist for the Carers (Recognition and Services) Act 1995.

Developments in the self-organisation of users of welfare services illustrate much diversity amongst user groups (Barnes, 1997). The self-help organisations enable previously unconsulted groups to have their voices heard and make their views known. Barnes argues that these organisations are not solely concerned with the redistribution of material goods or with changing the balance of power, 'they are also seeking to change the nature of the discourse within which notions of age, disability and mental disorder are constructed' (ibid., p. 70). Literature on user empowerment and self-help for older people is less in evidence, although there have been some initiatives to give older people a voice in community care (Thornton and Tozer, 1995; Jack, 1995; Cormie, 1999; Carter and Beresford, 2000).

Links can be made to the material in the previous chapter. There was material in Chapter 6 on the importance of social networks and the concept of social capital was introduced. Clearly, self-help groups and user-organisations are a means to helping people develop social networks and expand their social capital. Community development has also been a means of doing this and we turn to this next.

Community development and community care

Community care takes place within a community context and a useful avenue to explore in this respect is the connection between user involvement and community development. Historically, many users have been segregated from the general population and socially excluded from mainstream society. User empowerment needs to be considered not only in terms of individual empowerment but also from the perspective of collective empowerment, empowerment to relate to the wider community and empowerment as part of the wider community (Barr *et al.*, 1997).

Identifying opportunities for empowerment was made difficult by the individualistic interpretation of community care during the 1990s. Earlier chapters have noted the process whereby a person is assessed against 'eligibility criteria'. Individuals who meet these criteria receive a service. The structures were set up to target individuals in 'greatest need'. In the Department of Health's guidance for practitioners on the community care changes (DoH, 1991b), there was no mention of a community approach. The emphasis was on setting up individual care management with individual assessment, care plans and packages of care. Thus, discussions of empowerment frequently just related to 'individual' empowerment and did not consider the other collective aspects. The possibilities provided by such individual 'empowerment' were inevitably narrow and limited.

Techniques and skills of community development play a part in the process of empowerment. The philosophy of community development focuses on people who are excluded or oppressed, the structural causes of exclusion or oppression, collective social change, high levels of participation and the process of change. The strategies and skills employed in community development have been drawn on a great deal in health promotion work and there are advocates for them in other areas of health work (Clarke, 1998). Sometimes the language or 'capacity building' is used as a way of describing the outcomes of this sort of work.

So much community care is provided within the community by family, friends and neighbours that it is not sensible to ignore the contribution of community work practice and skills to the total picture. I have argued elsewhere and in more detail that 'there needs to be a strategy that links community care into the strengths and weaknesses of the local community, the support networks and the lack of support networks, the churches, the community groups, the friendship patterns' (Sharkey, 2000a). There are possibilities of linking community development and community care through the user-empowerment rhetoric of the community care changes that in turn can be linked to the participatory traditions of community work.

We have seen that the development and growth of self-help groups, user groups and new social movements was one of the most interesting and inspiring aspects of the 1980s and the 1990s. This bottom-up growth raises the question of whether community care practitioners can link up with such groups in a way that is constructive and neither patronising nor colonising (that is, the practitioners should not take over). Are there ways in which practitioners can move away from their individualistic orientation towards greater user involvement and a more collective approach? The rhetoric of empowerment and user involvement used by agencies and the Department of Health can be drawn on to develop approaches that are more collective and participatory in nature. It continues to be the case that service-user involvement and participation is extolled in much government guidance.

Barr *et al.* (1997) list the values that community care and community development have in common: empowerment, social inclusion, partnership, needs-led approaches, and participation. They outline four ways in which community development overlaps with user involvement and thus has a role to play in community care:

- *Collective user influence on service provision*. This concerns the level of control and influence users and carers have over the services they use. The emphasis here is on self-advocacy and empowerment. Suggested examples range from community advisory committees to full user control of the service.

- *Collective policy planning influence.* This concerns the influence users and carers have over the policy framework that determines the services they receive. Examples here are the care forums that have been introduced by a number of authorities.
- *Community service provision.* This is service provision by users/carers on their own or by other community organisations.
- *Supportive communities.* The focus here is on changes and developments within neighbourhoods to create more favourable conditions for community care users or carers to become integrated into community life. Examples include good neighbour schemes, volunteering, circles of support and community education.

It is through the user-empowerment aspects of the community care changes that a link can be made to collective empowerment of care users and carers as communities of interest and to the role neighbourhoods can play in supporting community care. There is clearly a gap between rhetoric and reality in respect to user empowerment and community development can help to bridge this gap. Barr *et al.* (ibid., p. 141) present a number of case studies and argue that 'The case studies illustrate that community development is an approach which takes forward user involvement and participation and seeks to make clear links between care user groups and the society of which they are a part'. They urge that a stronger connection be made between community care and community development, saying that health and welfare professionals have embraced the language of concepts such as empowerment, participation and anti-discriminatory practice but have continued to pursue an individualistic approach to assessment and care planning. 'This myopia constrains the application of these concepts which find their real potential in collective action by and with communities to meet their own needs and pursue more relevant and effective services' (ibid., p. 150).

In a later study called *Caring Communities*, Barr *et al.* (2001) make a further contribution to the debate on how community development approaches to community care can promote participative, inclusive and supportive communities. This was a three-year action-research project on the impact of a community development approach to community care. There was a focus on four sites in Scotland and all four provided evidence of the benefits that community development approaches can offer in the context of community care.

If community care is to be truly empowering, it must empower people beyond their role as services users and carers. The aim is that previously marginalised and excluded people should become part of the local community and participate in it (Barnes, 1997). Barnes argues that the concept of community care needs to be widened to include community participation. If this is to be achieved 'It has to involve enabling people to participate in decision making processes about services, and in social, economic and political life more broadly' (ibid., p. 172).

A wider interpretation of community care is needed rather than a narrowing down to individual care packages. With this wider vision, it is possible to draw on the real strengths of users/carers to ensure that they make an effective contribution to the well-being of society. Community work approaches give ideas on how this wider vision can be achieved by practitioners. Practitioners of preventive healthcare have been at the front of the field in recognising the importance of community work in achieving a positive change in health at the local level (DoH, 1999b).

Models of empowerment

So far this chapter has considered government policy in relation to empowerment and then the influence on practice of the idea of independent living, the social model, normalisation, and the user movement. The practice of community development has also exerted some influence and could be taken further.

Most people claim to be in favour of empowerment, but is it simply the case that it is a contested term and different people apply different meanings to it? One way of exploring this is to think in terms of models of empowerment. One such model is that of the consumer who has a greater choice of services. This is called the consumerist model. An alternative model is where the user has greater control over the services and this can be called the democratic model (Beresford and Croft, 1993; Robson *et al.*, 1997; Carter and Beresford, 2000).

The consumerist model views users as consumers. Governments of the 1980s and the early 1990s aimed to impose market ideas on public service provision, and consumerism in the public services meant bringing market principles to bear. A key element of the consumerist approach to public services is that the user has more choice because of the greater range of services on offer. The purchaser/provider split is seen as central to this. The user has more and clearer information on the services available and who the services are for. Representation and advocacy may be available for users. There is access to a complaints procedure. In this model these are all key factors in making the services more responsive to users as consumers.

While the consumerist model has been associated with New Right politics and ideas, the democratic model has been associated with the emergence of disabled people's organisations, self-advocacy and service users' organisations and movements (Croft and Beresford, 1999). Central to the democratic model is the idea of users having a greater say in and control over services as well as greater choice. This model draws on traditions of community work and community action, which have always strongly emphasised power and participation issues. The consumerist model emphasises information for users and user involvement but is not really concerned with user power. Customers in a shop can choose between the selection of products on display and have a certain choice between different shops, but they do not determine what is put on the shelf, that is, they have very little power over the selection of products from which to choose.

'Choice' became an increasingly used work in relation to health and social care provision during the early years of the new century. Governments wanted to increase choice for patients and service users. It could usually be seen within the consumerist model and the points about consumerism in a general sense made in the previous paragraph can be applied to consumerism within the health and welfare services. Choice is limited. For example, an older person may be able to choose between three day centres, but that is as far as it goes. The democratic model would raise issues about users having a say in whether they want day centres, where the day centres should be located, what goes on in them and how decisions are taken within them. The consumerist model lacks this dimension of power over what is provided and how it is provided.

So far, two models of empowerment have been described. In reality it may be more helpful to think in terms of a 'ladder of empowerment' with a succession of steps or stages. In their training pack on community care and community development, Barr et al. (1997, p. 21) describe the stages shown in Box 7.4.

Box 7.4   A ladder of empowerment

'Manipulation – Creating an illusion of participation resulting in disempowerment.
Informing – Telling people what is planned.
Consultation – Offering options and listening to feedback.
Deciding Together – Encouraging others to provide additional ideas and join in deciding the best way forward.
Acting Together – Deciding together and forming partnerships to act.

Supporting Independent Community Interests – Helping others to do what they want.'

If you are a practitioner then try to apply the above ladder to a situation or situations with which you are involved.

Some of the ideas discussed earlier in the chapter can be applied to the ladder in Box 7.4. It was noted earlier that disability groups campaigned for many years for direct payments to be made to them so that they could pay for their own care. This sprang from the independent living movement for people with physical disabilities. Schemes such as this are close to 'supporting independent community interests'. As you move to the other end of the ladder, users have less and less control over the services on offer and less and less say in how they are provided.

Social exclusion and regeneration

Chapter 1 introduced the notion of social exclusion in relation to community care. It also stressed the need for practitioners to make connections between personal problems and the wider structural issues such as poverty or inadequate housing. This section returns to that theme by looking at social exclusion and regeneration. Socially excluded people have often been geographically concentrated in certain areas and so area-based regeneration policies have often been a key part of the policy response.

Tackling social exclusion has been a major theme of New Labour policies before and since the 1997 election and social exclusion is now part of the common currency of debates about social policy in the United Kingdom. The Social Exclusion Unit (SEU), was set up in 1997 and was based in the Cabinet Office and reported directly to the Prime Minister on how to 'develop integrated and sustainable approaches to the worst housing estates, including crime, drugs, unemployment, community breakdown, and bad schools, etc.' (SEU, 1998). The SEU's remit is confined to England, although similar policies have been adopted in the rest of the United Kingdom.

In the book *Understanding Social Exclusion*, Hills argues that one of the advantages of looking at social exclusion is that it gives attention to aspects of deprivation which go beyond cash and material living standards (Hills, 2002, p. 242). The concept can include the dynamics of why some groups (such as older people or people with mental health problems) may be marginalised. Resolving this requires the development of closer links between community care developments and social exclusion policies (Sharkey, 2000b). This view is echoed in a report by the Social Exclusion Unit in 2004 which said, 'Community care policies need to be broadened to embrace more effectively the social exclusion agenda. While the extent of change in this policy area has been extensive over the past decade, there is a case for widening the scope of this work and extending the ambitions of care in the community' (SEU, 2004b, p. 8). In 2004, this same report for the Social Exclusion Unit examined the impact of government policy on social exclusion among older people. It included an outline of the gains made by the reforms in community care, notably in helping to maintain very dependent older people in their own homes for longer periods. However, it noted the limitations of the impact of community care policies on the social exclusion of older people. It summarised these as:

- limitations of low-level preventive work with older people;
- continuing problems in maximising user-involvement and empowerment;
- problem of continuing focus on survival needs to the detriment of inclusion of older people into mainstream activities;
- limited integration of community care with community development;
- continuing difficulties faced by marginalized groups such as those with mental health needs, black and minority ethnic elders, and carers.' (2004b, p. 65)

The report examined the possibility of refocusing the community care debate around social inclusion issues and argues in the conclusion that 'promoting social inclusion is an integral part of community care practice' (ibid., p. 89). A later report from the social exclusion unit (SEU, 2006) stressed the 'multiple exclusion' of many older people. It advocated a Sure Start service for older people and cross-government action to tackle social exclusion in this age group.

Similarly in 2003 the Social Exclusion Unit were asked to consider what was needed to reduce social exclusion among adults with mental health problems. The ensuing report (SEU, 2004a) focused on what more could be done to assist people with mental health problems to enter and retain work and have the same opportunities for social participation and access to services as the general population.

Within the overall policies on social exclusion there has been an emphasis on neighbourhood renewal or neighbourhood regeneration. In poor areas (or areas particularly identified as in need of regeneration), there are often a large number of community care concerns. This might be because there are high concentrations of people with mental health problems or drug/alcohol problems. Problems that affect whole communities are not best responded to by individualistic responses by health and social care services. During the

1980s and the early 1990s, the emphasis of regeneration was on economic objectives and the role of the private sector. Regeneration policies and approaches since the mid-1990s, however, have clearly included a social dimension (SEU, 1998). These government policies have an important role to play in developing a sensible way forward in community care. Community care workers can help by moving on from 'picking up the pieces' in a poor area to helping the whole community and its people to move forward, improve the quality of their lives and have some say over the future of their area.

An individualistic approach is a highly inadequate response by itself and other approaches are required. As Davey (1999, p. 37) has written, 'People who are seriously disadvantaged in society rarely have single problems – they have multiple interlocking problems.... Empowerment must address all their problems together if it is to be meaningful.' A broad approach, tackling the interlocking problems and looking for the common causes, is essential.

A problem that many of those involved in regeneration projects have stressed is that the mainstream public services in poor neighbourhoods are frequently ineffective (SEU, 1998, p 10). In spite of numerous demands for programmes to be 'bent' towards the needs of poor areas, there is little evidence that this happens (ibid., p. 38). The requirement here is for health and social care agencies to bend their provision towards poor areas and use their resources in an imaginative way. There is a need to analyse the problems, understand what the government is trying to do with area-based projects and work with the policies rather than against them. A key point is that the mainstream welfare services and indeed societal structures can encourage and create exclusion or inclusion. As Parkinson (1998, p. 34) states, 'Explicit urban strategies can make a difference, but mainstream programmes make a greater one'. Thus mainstream policies and practices within health and social work need to change.

The need for the involvement of local people and for community development to be a central part of the regeneration strategy is frequently stressed. For example, 'The most powerful resource in turning around neighbourhoods should be the community itself. Community involvement can take many forms: formal volunteering; helping a neighbour; taking part in a community organisation. It can have the triple benefit of getting things done that need to be, fostering community links and building the skills, self-esteem and networks of those who give their time' (SEU, 1998, p. 68). It is important for workers in mainstream programmes such as community care to back the policies and practices of the local regeneration strategy. It is acknowledged that regeneration requires local participation to be successful, so it follows that community care activities must also be participatory and collective.

Mutual aid and self-help are seen as crucial to addressing the issues of poverty, exclusion and regeneration (Burns and Taylor, 1998). The Labour government has placed some emphasis on communitarian ideas and mutual aid. Community work strategies and skills have much to offer in relation to tackling social exclusion and community work has a history of both tackling social divisions and working to empower people (Mayo, 1998).

Regeneration strategies are frequently concerned with issues of direct interest to community care service users. A housing strategy needs to have supported housing as a central part of its agenda. An employment strategy needs to have policies to assist disabled people enter the job market. Hence the importance of community care users and workers being involved directly and closely in the development of local policy.

Practice issues

As an exercise, if you are a practitioner, reflect on a situation in which you are involved - this could be to do with an individual, a group or the wider community. Try to place that situation on the ladder of user involvement prescribed in Box 7.4. What are some of the blockages to moving to a position of greater user empowerment on the ladder? Can those blockages be removed?

Service users often need information in order to challenge decisions made about them. A range of ways in which decisions on care management can be challenged are given at the end of Chapter 4. Practitioners need to be knowledgeable about these mechanisms in order to provide information at appropriate times. Practitioners should also find out which user groups are operating in their area of work and consider the ways in which support might be given. Care should be taken to act sensitively and to avoid the 'I know best' attitude exhibited by some workers.

In this chapter it is argued that there was more rhetoric than reality about user empowerment in the community care changes. Other changes and influences have, however, encouraged empowerment in different ways and the influence of the independent living movement, the social model of disability, normalisation, the user movement, and community work has been discussed. All have provided some vision, progress and encouragement when other pressures have forced practice into an individualistic and bureaucratic mode. It has been further argued that policies on social exclusion and regeneration offer opportunities for practitioners to engage in the wider debates and practices (focusing on participation, involvement and change) that are evolving. To avoid this would be to miss the opportunity presented by the Department of Health:

'More widely, social services can make an important contribution to wider local authority-led programmes to tackle the problems of homelessness, poor housing conditions, and social exclusion in deprived neighbour-hoods.' (DoH, 1998a, para. 6.23)

Ideas of anti-oppressive practice or anti-discriminatory practice are relevant to all sections of this book but perhaps especially in relation to this chapter. Thompson's (2006) PCS analysis provides a method for thinking about this. The P level stands for the personal level of thoughts, feelings, attitudes and actions. C stands for the cultural level of shared ways of seeing, thinking and doing. S relates to the structural level of society and the structures of power and oppression that exist in society (ibid., pp. 26–30). This provides a framework for relating individual and personal matters through to cultural issues and to the wider structural issues that we have referred to throughout the book.

There is a tendency to see empowerment in purely individual terms. While this is important, this chapter has stressed the desirability of collective empowerment strategies through involvement in self-help groups and community development. Practitioners need to consider how they can acquire skills that are relevant to this and be open to the possibilities it presents. Stewart (1993) argues for much more coverage in nursing education of working in partnership with self-help groups. Healthcare may too easily fall into the pattern of individual diagnosis and the prescription of drugs in cases where mutual support may be more relevant and helpful.

Priestley (1999) has looked at the Derbyshire Integrated Living Scheme in the context of the wider user movement and national and international policies and developments. Practitioners need to try to make the same connections between local work and wider national and international developments. A quotation from Priestley's book is worth reflecting on in this respect: 'There are many battles to be won and the sheer scale of those which remain requires the maintenance of a visionary agenda for the liberation of disabled people. As the example of disabled people's organisations in Derbyshire shows, acting locally and thinking globally has proved to be good maxim for action' (ibid., p. 226).

Further reading

Swain, J., French, S., Barnes, C. and Thomas, C. (2004) *Disabling Barriers – Enabling Environments* 2nd edn ((London: Sage). This textbook on disability studies has a variety of chapters examining particularly aspects of the social model of disability.

Thompson, N. (2006) *Anti-Discriminatory Practice*, 4th edn (London: Palgrave). Thompson, N. (2003) *Promoting Equality*, 2nd edn (London: Palgrave). Both books provides a framework for understanding discrimination, oppression and social divisions.

Journals that have debated in much more detail some of the issues relating to disability contained in this chapter are *Disability and Society*, the *British Journal of Learning Disabilities* and the *Journal of Applied Research in Intellectual Disabilities*.

World Wide Web sites

The British Council of Disabled People was set up in 1981 and is an umbrella organisation representing over 120 disabled people's groups. Its web site is at www.bcodp.org.uk

The website of the National Centre for Independent Living is designed to be a resource on independent living and direct payments for disabled people and others working in the field and can be found at http://www.ncil.org.uk

CHAPTER 8

Adult Abuse and Community Care

Chapter summary

This chapter discusses:

- Elder abuse as a developing social problem in the United Kingdom.
- Some links between adult abuse, child abuse and domestic violence.
- Definitions and prevalence of abuse.
- Institutional abuse.
- The legal context of abuse.
- The wider context.
- Intervention and practice.

Introduction

The abuse of adults brings together many of the topics discussed in this book. Interdisciplinary approaches, links to assessment and care management, empowerment, informal carers and networks of care – all of these themes of previous chapters are important when considering the abuse of adults.

One of the big omissions in the 1989 White Paper (DoH, 1989a) and the NHS&CC Act 1990, was the subject of adult abuse. A year after the community care legislation was passed, Virginia Bottomley (then Junior Minister of Health) stated on television that 'I don't frankly think that abuse of the elderly is a major issue, thank goodness, in our society' ('Newsnight', BBC2, 4 June 1991). This lack of government acknowledgement of elder and adult abuse helps to explain why it was ignored during the development of legislation and policy for adults. However, the growing evidence of its prevalence and increasing concern about it makes it central to considerations of community care. This chapter starts with a particular focus on elder abuse and the development of the issue. There is then an exploration of the connections between adult abuse, child abuse and domestic violence.

This is followed by comment on the definition of abuse, types of abuse, their prevalence and the settings in which they occur. Intervention needs to be grounded in the current legal context and take account of social divisions such as ageism, sexism and disablism. This wider context within which abuse takes place is considered and, as usual, the chapter finishes by looking at some issues in relation to practice.

The development of elder abuse as a social problem

The topic of abuse is complicated by a plethora of definitional and conceptual differences. What may be considered as abuse by one generation or one society may not be seen as such by another. Both adult abuse and child abuse are socially constructed. How abuse is seen reflects the values and views of a particular time and a particular culture. It is therefore not easy to define, although any one society at any one time may define it for the purposes of intervention and action against it.

There are both similarities and differences between domestic violence, child abuse, elder abuse and the abuse of other vulnerable adults. It is important to search for both of those aspects. Child abuse is readily identifiable as an issue of concern or a social problem and has been since the Maria Colwell inquiry of the early 1970s. Domestic violence was largely neglected by the health and welfare services until it was brought to their attention by the women's movement and the refuge movement. The abuse of people with disabilities and with mental health problems has been neglected, and there is little literature, media coverage or research to draw on. Elder abuse has emerged as a social problem since the late 1980s (Penhale and Kingston, 1995, p. 226; Manthorpe, 1999). Box 8.1 picks out some of the key events and research that led to the gradual acknowledgement of elder abuse as a social problem.

Box 8.1   The development of elder abuse in the UK as a social problem

1960s

- Institutional abuse was taken seriously as a result of the writing of people such as Townsend (1962) and Robb (1967).

1970s

- Social worker Mervyn Eastman, using his own records and other contacts and information, drew attention to the issue in the mid-1970s. Journalists and editors gave the unfortunate (and unacceptable) label of 'granny bashing' to the phenomenon.

1980s

- The voluntary organisation Age Concern played an important role in keeping the issue on the agenda and in 1984 it published *Old Age Abuse* by Eastman. This was followed in 1986 by *The Law and Vulnerable Elderly People* (Age Concern, 1986), which included coverage of abuse.
- The problem was identified in the United Kingdom and North America at about the same time, but while it received attention as a policy and practice issue in the United States, the United Kingdom was slow to respond. In the United States, Pillemer and Wolf's *Elder Abuse* (1986) was regarded as a seminal work. The topic maintained a high profile and most US states now have clear legislation in relation to elder abuse.
- In 1988, a British Geriatric Society conference drew together practitioners and stimulated debate. The conference report suggested that 10 per cent of older people were victims of abuse (Bennett *et al.*, 1997, p. 13).

1990s

- The publication of a 1992 study on the prevalence of elder abuse in the United Kingdom promoted further debate (Ogg and Bennett, 1992).
- Practice guidance to local authorities, *No Longer Afraid* (DoH, 1993), was published when the authorities were grappling with the implementation of the community care changes. However, it was not integral to those changes. No money was allocated to support the guidance and no action was taken against local authorities that failed to heed the guidance. *No Longer Afraid* advocated that care management principles be applied to situations of abuse. While it recommended a strong interagency approach, it was addressed only to social service authorities and not to other statutory bodies such as health authorities (Ambache, 1997).
- A number of other works (many of which are mentioned in this chapter) published in the 1990s helped to raise the profile of the issue.
- The organisation Action on Elder Abuse was formed in 1993 and has since played an important role in breaking the taboo on examining and discussing the issue. It set up a national telephone helpline in 1997.
- A campaign by *Community Care* magazine in 1993 highlighted the issue for social work practitioners.
- Consultation papers by the English Law Commission and the Scottish Law Commission on vulnerable adults were published during the early 1990s and these triggered debate on the weakness of legislation in this area.
- At the local level, most social service authorities drew up and adopted policies and procedures relating to elder abuse during the 1990s, usually in

consultation with other agencies such as health authorities. These documents provided valuable guidelines for practitioners. However, these policies varied from area to area so there was uneven development. There remained a need for a national strategy and a national lead.

- In December 1997, the government published the Green Paper *Who Decides?* (Lord Chancellor's Department, 1997), containing the package of proposals relating to England and Wales that had been put together by the Law Commission in 1995. Among the proposals were the modernisation of laws relating to mental incapacity, and the introduction of new powers to enable social workers to intervene to protect vulnerable adults such as elderly people, those with serious physical illnesses and those incapable of making their own decisions.
- In 1998 the 'Practitioner Alliance Against Abuse of Vulnerable Adults' was set up in order to bring practitioners together and give them a voice in the ongoing debate.

2000s

- In 2000, *No Secrets* (DoH, 2000a) in England and *In Safe Hands* (National Assembly for Wales, 2000a) in Wales gave guidance on developing and implementing multi-agency procedures to protect vulnerable adults from abuse. Each authority now has these procedures in place. New laws were therefore not brought in and the policies applied to 'all' vulnerable adults and not just older people. By this stage it could be argued that there was some acknowledgement of elder abuse as a social problem – this was within the wider context of the abuse of all vulnerable adults.
- In 2000, the Adults with Incapacity (Scotland) Act 2000 introduced a new structure of supporting people who had not the capacity to make decisions for themselves.
- The Care Standards Act 2000 provided for the regulation and inspection of care services in England and Wales. This was particularly in response to criticisms of the poor standards in some residential homes and criticisms of previous inspection systems.
- The Health & Social Care Act 2003 created new structures for the regulation of health and social care provision in England and Wales.
- In 2004, The House of Commons Health Committee produced a report on elder abuse.
- In 2004, the Pova list was started. The Care Standards Act 2000 made provision for a list to be established of individuals judged to be unsuitable to work with vulnerable adults. This was the Protection of Vulnerable Adults (POVA) list. It applied to England and Wales. The POVA list is supposed to be a workforce ban on people who have abused or mistreated vulnerable adults in the past.

- The Domestic Violence, Crime and Victims Act 2004 introduced a new offence of familial homicide where the death of a child or vulnerable person is caused by a member of the household.
- The Mental Capacity Act 2005 was passed, with a view to implementation in 2007. It covered England and Wales and it governed decision-making on behalf of adults, in cases in which they lose mental capacity at some point in their lives or in which the incapacitating condition has been present since birth. The Act clarified a number of legal uncertainties and reforms and updated the law where decisions need to be made on behalf of others.

The chronology in Box 8.1 serves to indicate some acknowledgement over the years of elder abuse as a 'social problem'. Since the turn of the century it has been acknowledged by governments within the more generic context of 'vulnerable adults'. However, as a topic it continues to struggle to gain the attention it merits. It is an intriguing issue as to how the abuse of adults has received so little attention in comparison to the abuse of children over the past thirty years. The 2004 *House of Commons Health Committee Report on Elder Abuse* started by contrasting the fact that many people would be familiar with the details of Victoria Climbié, who was tortured and murdered in the care of a relative but that few would know about Margaret Panting, a 78-year-old woman from Sheffield who died after suffering great cruelty while she was living with her relatives. The report writes,

'After her death in 2001, a post-mortem found 49 injuries on her body including cuts probably made by a razor blade and cigarette burns. She had moved from sheltered accommodation to her son-in-law's home – five weeks later she was dead. But as the cause of Margaret Panting's death could not be established, no one was ever charged. An inquest in 2002 recorded an open verdict.' (HoC, 2004, para. 1)

Adult abuse, child abuse and domestic violence

Since the 1970s, in the United Kingdom there has been considerable publicity about and reports, legislation and research on child abuse, from which it may be possible to draw some lessons that are applicable to elder abuse. In child protection, there is a range of orders under the Children Act 1989 (in Scotland the Children (Scotland) Act 1995) that can be called on. These include powers to investigate and emergency protection orders, posing the question as to whether similar orders might be appropriate in the case of vulnerable adults.

It is easy to focus on the lack of legislation and procedures for adults in contrast with the numerous measures to protect children and to assume automatically that similar legislation would be helpful. Social work in child care has become dominated by child protection work and Eastman (1999) poses the question of whether social work with adults would become dominated by investigative work if there was a stronger legal framework. If resources were tight, would other aspects of social work with adults become neglected? Eastman therefore argues that there is a case for the police dealing with this investigative work. Perry (2004) has also questioned why the implementation of *No Secrets* (DoH, 2000a) was not given to the police.

Good interprofessional working in child protection has in the past been helped and fostered by 'area child protection committees'. The idea has been taken up in the area of adult protection. *No Secrets* asked local councils and partner agencies to consider establishing 'adult protection commit-tees' (DoH, 2000a). The intention of these was to determine local policies, coordinate activity between agencies, facilitate joint training, and monitor and review progress.

There is a wealth of experience in child protection work on how to deal with abuse when it is revealed or suspected. With both groups, this work requires skill and sensitivity. Information can be given to staff at any time, for example at a day centre or alone with a home care worker. It is essential for all workers to have some idea of how to respond. No worker can promise confidentiality in this situation and they need to make it clear that they are obliged to inform their line manager.

There are distinct differences between child protection work and adult protection work in the sense that adults are deemed to be competent to make decisions and therefore have a clear right to self-determination and choice. In the *No Secrets* guidance, advocates of inter-agency adult protec-tion work are to 'act in a way which supports the rights of the individual to lead an independent life based on self-determination and personal choice' (DoH, 2000a, p. 21). The guidance gives a reminder that such a right to self-determination will involve risk. The guidance also indicates the need to 'recognise people who are unable to take their own decisions and/or to protect themselves, their assets and bodily integrity' (ibid.).

In relation to domestic violence, there is a need to see victims of domestic violence within the wider context of community care and to investigate any possible links between domestic violence and other forms of abuse. What should be the same and what different in respect of policies, procedures and intervention? Some elder abuse is the continuation of abuse from earlier years and yet relatively few links have been made between the two areas of study. As McCreadie (1996, p. 17) wrote, 'the domestic violence literature

has barely concerned itself with older people and the elder abuse literature has barely concerned itself with domestic violence'.

Connections have been made and a useful book by Kingston and Penhale
(1995) drew out some of these. Biggs *et al.* (1995, p. 110) argue that
domestic violence intervention models tend to stress crisis intervention
services, emergency refuges, support groups, counselling facilities and legal
expertise. The emphasis is on providing immediate protection once the
abuse is identified. It is argued that this has contrasted with the approach to
other forms of adult abuse, where there has often been a reluctance to act.
Police forces have been increasingly encouraged to treat domestic abuse as
a crime but this is has been slower to develop in other areas of adult abuse.

It should be clear that abuse is not a straightforward problem for which
there are easy answers or solutions. It is far easier to provide a list of
questions on the topic that are largely unresolved. Box 8.2 lists some of these.

Box 8.2   Questions for debate

- What do child abuse, domestic abuse and adult abuse have in common and
  what is different?
- If abuse can occur throughout the life cycle, what is the justification for
  categorisation by age? (Slater, 1999)
- Are there common roots, explanations and interventions, or should we be
  cautious of drawing such links?
- When do poor levels of hygiene, healthcare and safety become neglect and
  what is the limitation on individual liberty and self-determination to choose to
  live as they wish?
- At what point does verbal aggression become psychological abuse?
- Do we need a stronger legislative framework in relation to adult abuse?
- Should the lead workers investigating the abuse of adults be social workers or
  the police? (Eastman, 1999)

It is clear that there are many questions and most of them stimulate
debate rather than clear answers.

Definitions and prevalence

In the previous section we saw that there are many 'questions for debate' in
this area of adult abuse. There is also much discussion about some of the

definitions of key terms such as abuse, capacity and vulnerable. These are quite contested terms and open for discussion and debate.

It was noted in Box 8.1 that *No Secrets* in England and *In Safe Hands* in Wales required local authorities to develop multi-agency policies and procedures to protect vulnerable adults from abuse (DoH, 2000a: National Assembly for Wales, 2000a). According to *No Secrets*, a vulnerable person is someone, 'who is or may be in need of community care services by reason of mental or other disability, age or illness; and who is or may be unable to take care of him or herself, or unable to protect him or herself against significant harm or exploitation' (DoH, 2000a, para. 2.3). This definition has achieved some currency. Clearly, it applies to all adults and not just older people. One could argue that users and potential service users are not the only vulnerable people (HoC, 2004). Refugees and asylum-seekers, for example, may be particularly vulnerable and this may largely be due to the societal structures they have come from and the societal structures within which they now live (Williams, 2004b). The definition does not lend itself to those situations where societal and environmental factors create vulnerability.

People who are not able to make their own decisions are described as lacking in 'capacity'. This lack of capacity may be due to, for example, an illness such as dementia or a brain injury or mental health problems. This is an area that we will return to later in the chapter. Capacity is not easy to define and sometimes not easy to determine.

There are debates about the definition of abuse. In England, the *No Secrets* guidance defined abuse as 'a violation of an individual's human and civil rights by any other person or persons' (DoH, 2000a, p. 9). It gave six categories of abuse that were physical, sexual, psychological, financial, neglect and discriminatory abuse. Again this definition and categorisation could be contested. The main point to be made is that this is an area where the terms vulnerable, capacity and abuse are used, linked and inter-twined. While there may be 'working definitions' there is much debate and uncertainty about the terms.

Prevalence of abuse is not easy to determine for a number of reasons. First, there are debates about the definition of abuse. Second, abuse is bound to be hidden to a large extent because it is not something that people readily talk about. Third, measuring abuse is complicated because abuse is a complex phenomenon which takes different forms, occurs in different settings and takes place in various kinds of relationship.

The first indication of the scale of the problem in the United Kingdom was provided by Ogg and Bennett (1992), who reported on the results of structured interviews with 593 people aged 65 and over. Excluded were older people in institutions and those who were too ill or disabled to participate, and this may have concealed the true extent of abuse. Fifty people reported some kind of abuse. Of these, nine reported physical abuse, nine financial abuse and 32 verbal abuse. Adult members of households in regular contact with a person of pensionable age were asked if they had ever abused an older person. Of the 1,366 questioned, 10 per cent admitted to verbal abuse and 1 per cent acknowledged physical abuse (ibid.). While limited in nature, this study did demonstrate that there was a serious problem.

In 2004, the Health Committee of the House of Commons wrote, 'The figure of at least half a million people experiencing some form of abuse at any point in time appears to offer the only estimate that is currently available' (HoC, 2004, para 31). The Committee mentioned a survey of community and district nurses, commissioned by the Community and District Nursing Association in 2003, which had indicated that the vast majority of respondents encountered elder abuse at work (88 per cent). In 12 per cent of cases this was on a monthly, or more frequent basis (HoC, 2004, para. 21).

The charity Action on Elder Abuse has run a helpline and has done an analysis of the nearly 7,000 calls to it since 1997 (AEA, 2004). Two-thirds of the calls to the helpline related to abuse in the victim's home. Nearly a quarter of callers complained of abuses in care homes, where less than 5 per cent of older people live. In 46 per cent of cases, the alleged abuser was related to their victim, usually a son or daughter (50 per cent of these) or partner (23 per cent). Paid workers were blamed in one-third of calls. The main forms of abuse were psychological (34 per cent), financial (20 per cent) and physical (19 per cent). Sixty-seven per cent of those who were reported suffering abuse were women and 22 per cent were men. The remaining 11 per cent were accounted for by men and women facing abuse at the same time.

While elder abuse has been neglected, the abuse of other vulnerable adults has received even less attention. Little is known, for example, about the abuse of people with mental health problems. It is of course hard to obtain reliable figures because abuse is shrouded in secrecy. With regard to people with learning difficulties, in a study by Brown and colleagues at the University of Kent in the early 1990s, it is estimated that at that time there were around 1,200 new cases each year of the sexual abuse of adults with learning difficulties in England and Wales (Craft, 1996). The lesson here for practitioners is that they should be alert to the possibility that it is taking place.

Some older people and other vulnerable adults suffer harassment from strangers in the community. 'Community harassment' or 'stranger abuse' is little researched, but in some city areas older people are afraid to leave their houses and some individuals have suffered considerable abuse and persecution (Biggs *et al.*, 1995, p. 74). Pritchard (1995, p. 32) has written of the growing concern about older people being abused by young people in their communities, and of the growing problem of drug abuse in the United Kingdom and the link between this and the abuse of elders. With adults from ethnic minority groups there can be an element of racism in abuse (Biggs, 1996). Perry has written about 'hate crime' against people with learning disabilities (2004). Individualised care management is an inappropriate response to these community problems and there is a need, as stressed in Chapter 7, for links to neighbourhood regeneration policies and policies that deal with discrimination and social exclusion.

Institutional abuse

The 1993 DoH guidelines concentrated on abuse in the home. This was rather strange given that scandals about abuse in institutions go back some decades. The practice of care in the community was given particular impetus by the abuse, neglect and shameful conditions revealed by a succession of hospital inquiries (concerning people with learning difficulties and mental health problems). Earlier examples include Ely in 1968, South Ockenden in 1969, Farleigh in 1970 and Whittingham in 1971. Further inquiries took place in the late 1970s, including that into Normansfield Hospital in 1978.

Given this history, it is important to consider institutional settings, such as day care facilities, residential homes, nursing homes and hospitals (Clough, 1996). People often enter these settings so that they can be cared for and kept safe, but sadly they may still find themselves victims of abuse. Concern about institutional abuse played a part in the move towards community care. McCreadie (1996, p. 57) writes, 'As numerous enquiries into grave deficiencies in various areas of institutional care for all age groups have shown, abuse flourishes within a culture which allows it to be acceptable'. Pritchard (1996, pp. 114–15) notes that abuse can be perpetuated by a member of staff against a resident, a resident against a member of staff, a resident against another resident or an outsider against a resident. This can take place in any institutional setting. Section 48 of the NHS&CC Act 1990 required the setting up of inspection units within social service authorities to inspect all residential homes for adults. The local authority registration and inspection units and the health authority inspection units were part of the official machinery to safeguard against abuse in residential and nursing care. These units were required to inspect all institutions twice a year: one announced inspection and one unannounced. The 1997 Labour government wanted a greater level of independence for these inspection units.

Changes have taken place and in 2006 in England there is the Commission for Social Care Inspection that works in parallel with the Healthcare

Commission. In Scotland, there is the Commission for the Regulation of Care, accountable to the Scottish Parliament, and in Wales the Care Standards Inspectorate for Wales. In Northern Ireland, health and social care are integrated and inspection is by the Northern Ireland Health and Personal Services Regulation and Improvement Authority. Inspections are static snapshots taken at certain times and need to be part of a broader, continuous strategy. Such a strategy would include helping residents to voice their complaints. It would also encourage staff to bring problems into the open without fear of victimisation. The example in Box 8.3 illustrates the difficulty of this.

Box 8.3   Case study

In February 1997, the owner of an old people's home in Yorkshire was jailed for four years after pleading guilty to sexually assaulting women in his care who were suffering from senile dementia. The deputy matron, Judy Jones, risked her job to stop the owner forcing oral sex on elderly residents. She felt unable to raise the matter with the owner's wife, who ran the home, and she knew that if she went to the police it would simply be her word against his. With the help of the charity Public Concern at Work she developed a plan with other staff to protect the residents and obtain the necessary proof.

Public Concern at Work is a charity set up in 1994 and which aims to help employees expose serious malpractice in their workplace. A significant proportion of its work has been concerned with abuse in residential and nursing homes. It has a mission to ensure that concerns about serious malpractice are properly raised and addressed. It has called for legal protection for care home staff who expose abuse; a regulatory regime that actively encourages good practice in the sector; and for care homes to operate an open door policy for relatives and friends and to hold open days for the local community. What is needed is a system that enables concerns to be expressed and examined without victimisation. In a way this can be seen as building whistle-blowing into the system as a last resort. The Public Interest Disclosure Act 1998 goes some way towards providing legal protection for whistle-blowers.

Box 8.4   An example of whistle-blowing

In June, 2004, a senior ward sister was convicted of attempting to murder two elderly patients under her care. She was jailed for five years at Chester Crown

> Court. The hospital had a bed-blocking crisis and the nurse was seen by the court to be motivated by a desire to free up beds. In a statement, the Cheshire and Merseyside Strategic Health Authority said of the whistle-blowers, 'We are grateful to the hospital staff who first raised their concerns with the trust for bringing the matter to the attention of the police.' (*Guardian*, 19 June 2004)

If institutions are to be safe it is essential for them to remain open to ideas and inspections. When they become 'closed', abuse can become the norm. It is all too easy within a closed society for poor practice to deteriorate into unacceptable conduct. Lawson (1999) powerfully describes how as a trainee nurse in a hospital she felt she was being 'trained' into abusing patients by the experienced nurses with whom she worked. It was only some time later that she recognised that such practices were abusive. In an important and illuminating article drawing on public inquiries into institutional care, Wardhaugh and Wilding (1993) consider how institutions, organisations and staff who are supposedly committed to an ethic of care become 'corrupted' and abuse both their power and people in their care. They discuss how care becomes corrupted and how it can break down so that residents of institutions are put at risk. In order to avoid this 'corruption of care', there needs to be built-in safety mechanisms to prevent poor practice from taking hold. This involves a culture of openness, self-criticism, self-regulation, peer criticism, managerial support, supervision and control. What is required is a structure and environment where disclosure can take place naturally and where there are clear policies and procedures that make it easy to raise issues of concern, including abuse. Where mechanisms are in place there should be no need for whistle-blowing, but as a fall-back it would be useful to have procedures for whistle-blowing.

The legal context of abuse

Many feel that the national practice guidelines on the abuse of vulnerable adults are insufficient in themselves and there is a need for a change in the law. There is no clear legal framework for workers to intervene unless a person is 'mentally disordered'. Without the law on their side, professional workers are limited in what they can do. The carer can refuse to let professionals have access. The adult victim may refuse help. Clements, commenting on the guidance of 2000, has written that the processes set up, 'valuable as they may be, are no substitute for a statutory regime that enables social services (where material evidence of abuse exists) to gain access to and effectively protect vulnerable adults' (2004, p. 393).

Practitioners should bear in mind that there are laws against such crimes as assault, theft and rape and that these laws can be drawn on. There can, however, be some difficulties with making use of criminal law. The victim of abuse normally has to complain and be involved in the preparation of charges by the police. This can be distressing if a family member is involved. Furthermore, the police may be reluctant to pursue cases involving family disputes. There can also be a problem with older people and people with disabilities being taken seriously as victims of crime.

With regard to intervention, it is important for practitioners to be well informed about current legislation. Obtaining appropriate advice at the correct time from solicitors, law centres, specialist legal departments or charities is an important part of the process. Practitioners should be familiar with the relevant laws and how they might be used so that they can give knowledgeable advice when required. It is important to be able to draw on the law appropriately and at the correct time. Writing about elder abuse, Brammer (1996, p. 13) states that 'The challenge . . . calls on lawyers to be creative and use their imagination and skills in drawing on existing remedies from statute and common law and adapting these to respond to individual complaints'.

In the early 1990s, the English Law Commission engaged in a process of consultation on the need for changes to the law in respect of mental disability. One consultation paper was published in 1991 and three were published in 1993. The conclusions and recommendations were brought together in a fifth report, *Mental Incapacity* (Law Commission, 1995). This included a draft Mental Incapacity Bill. The original terms of reference were extended to other people who were vulnerable and in need of protection. The report is quite clear that reform is needed: 'The law as it now stands is unsystematic and full of glaring gaps. It does not rest on clear or modern foundations of principle. It has failed to keep up with developments in our understanding of the rights and needs of those with mental disability' (ibid., para. 1.1). Drawing on the Children Act 1989 and models for child protection, the proposals set out a clear framework for the investigation and assessment of situations of abuse (Brammer, 1996, p. 43). The Scottish Law Commission also reviewed the law in this area and published a report in 1995. The underlying principles of the Scottish approach were broadly similar to those of the English Law Commission (Lord Chancellor's Department, 1997).

The main recommendations of the English Law Commission were included in the Green Paper *Who Decides?* (ibid.). One recommendation was that social service authorities should have a new duty to investigate suspected neglect or abuse and be given the power to deal with the protection of people they believe to be at risk. As noted, this route of new legislation has not so far been followed. However the debate about it continues and there remain calls for a new, strong legislative framework in this area.

Going into the new century, the general approach adopted by government was to use a plethora of regulatory and inspectorial instruments to improve the quality of care and reduce abuse. These can be seen in the last section of Box 8.1, which also indicates that one aspect of actual legislation that did progress was concerned with 'mental incapacity'. In Scotland the Adults with Incapacity (Scotland) Act 2000 set a framework for decisions about such things as health, money and welfare. For England and Wales, the Mental Capacity Act was passed in 2005, with implementation in 2007. This legislation provides a statutory framework for people who may not be able to make their own decisions. This might be, for example, because of learning disability, an illness such as dementia or brain injury or mental health problems. The Act sets out who can take decisions, in which situations, and how they should go about this. Under this legislation, tougher maximum prison sentences of five years now exist for people found guilty of neglect or ill treatment of a person who lacks capacity. The overall intention of the legislation is to give a better framework to guide carers, families and professionals in decision-making if a person loses mental capacity.

The wider context

Most accounts of the causes of abuse have concentrated on the stress on carers and on family violence within dysfunctional families. Causes are always complex with many factors involved, but it is noticeable how much of the discussion on adult abuse has ignored wider societal issues. Causes are often described in a localised or narrow way and fail to acknowledge the wider structural issues at play. Thus, theories on carer stress and dysfunctional families have been very much to the fore. Most of the research on the causes of elder abuse has been conducted in the United States. McCreadie (1994, p. 16) summarised the two broad approaches as a function of, first, caregiving and, second, as an aspect of family violence. Similarly, while the SSI guidelines acknowledged that there were likely to be many different reasons why older people were abused, it was clear where the emphasis is: 'Carers under stress, or ill-equipped for the caring role, and carers who have been (and are still being) abused themselves, account for a proportion of cases. A history of poor family relationships is a reason for others. In some families, the power once exercised by the parent is also probably a factor' (DoH, 1993, p. 4).

These guidelines, like most of the literature on abuse, ignore the fact that abuse and harm takes place within an ageist, sexist and disablist society and fail to make connections with these structural factors of social division. It is important to bring social divisions to the forefront of discussion and put adult abuse into the context of an ageist, sexist and disablist society. Feminists and feminist theory have placed domestic violence in the context of male power and patriarchal attitudes and structures. Just as racism provides an explanatory backcloth to violence against black people (or heterosexism to violence against gay people), so one needs to see ageism, sexism and disablism as providing an explanatory backcloth to the harm and violence to older people (predominantly women) and disabled people in society (Biggs, 1996).

Ageism, for example, has a very considerable impact on how old people are viewed and treated (Thompson, 1995). Butler defines it as 'A process of systematic stereotyping and discrimination against people because they are old, just as racism and sexism accomplish this for skin colour and gender' (Butler, 1987, p. 22). This stereotyping and discrimination influences people's attitudes and behaviour. It can reduce the barriers to acts of abuse (Thompson, 1995). As a result of ageism in health and social care organisations, older people might receive a worse service than they should receive. It might be that acts of abuse are not taken as seriously as they would be if the person were younger.

Explanatory frameworks are important because they influence how practitioners see issues and what needs to be done. We have outlined frameworks that consider carer stress, dysfunctional families and wider structural issues. Dealing with individuals, there is a tendency for practitioners to be drawn to the more individual of family explanations. 'Carer stress' is probably viewed as the 'common sense' explanation of elder abuse. As the older person becomes more dependent, he or she makes more demands on the carer. The carer can no longer cope with these demands, resulting in abuse or neglect. This fits into the 'situational stress' theory (Penhale and Kingston, 1995, p. 192). If we accept this explanation, intervention will probably consist of relieving carer stress through some combination of respite service, day care and home care. However, such solutions tend to define the victim of abuse as the problem.

Much analysis of domestic violence looks to explanations connected to the power of men in society and within families. Violence is at the end of a continuum that maintains and asserts that power. Such an explanatory framework deriving from feminist writers, leads to theories of intervention that focus on escaping from the situation, removing the offender, and using the law to deal with the crime and protect the woman.

Whittaker (1995, p. 44) states 'Elder abuse, like other forms of abuse, must be seen as a crime against the person'. It is not satisfactory to try to explain it away compassionately as carer stress or the symptom of a dysfunctional family (DoH, 1993). It may be these things but it also a crime and it needs to be seen within the context of male violence to women within families and society (Dobash and Dobash, 1992). It should be located within the patriarchal family rather than the pathological family and it is important to avoid viewing the victim as the problem (Whittaker, 1995; Aitken and Griffin, 1996).

Practice issues

Confronted by a situation of possible adult abuse, practitioners sometimes feel inadequately prepared to cope. While the emotions are understandable, this is now less of a reason for inaction as there are guidelines, a body of knowledge and experienced practitioners who can give advice.

Working in situations of abuse requires considerable skill. It is also potentially very stressful, and as with any really difficult situation, it can produce in workers a range of emotions, such as helplessness, fear, blame, guilt, frustration, anger, denial and shame. There will be feelings of 'What could I have done?' or 'What should I have done next?' Thus, supervision and support are as important in this area of work as in others. This can help alleviate anxiety and assist in the consideration of all options.

Each local authority will have a multi-agency policy in relation to adult abuse. If you are practising as a health or social care worker then the obvious first step is to familiarise yourself with the policy for your area. Abuse situations almost always involve workers from different professions and good interdisciplinary working is essential.

Abuse and harm thrive on secrecy and they remain something of a taboo subject. Denial of it results in people and workers not recognising its existence or not addressing it. It is difficult to deal with and it is sometimes easier to deny what is in front of our eyes. The taboo needs to be broken at all levels because it is one of the factors that inhibits the disclosure of abuse by those abused, their relatives and health and social care workers. Breaking the taboo helps to break the secrecy, so this is a matter for practitioners to learn about, discuss and address in the workplace and the community.

Finally, it is necessary to avoid treating adult abuse as simply an individual concern in a domestic setting. It should be set in a community context and in the national context of discrimination and oppression.

Further reading

House of Commons Health Committee (2004) *Elder Abuse* (London: Stationery Office). This report gives a good overview of elder abuse. It can be viewed at www.parliament.the-stationery-office.co.uk

The Journal of Adult Protection, from Pavilion Publishing (Brighton), is published four times a year and is a way to keep up to date with issues and changes.

The organisation Action on Elder Abuse has several publications and leaflets that are useful for practitioners. It can be contacted at Action on Elder Abuse, Astral House, 1268 London Road, London SW16 4ER.

World Wide Web sites

Action on Elder Abuse has a website with information on the organisation itself and adult abuse: www.elderabuse.org.uk

Public Concern at Work (for 'whistle-blowers'): www.pcaw.co.uk

Women's Aid, the national charity working to end domestic violence against women and children: www.womensaid.org.uk

VoiceUK is a national charity supporting people with learning disabilities who have experienced crime or abuse: www.voiceuk.org.uk

International Network for the Prevention of Elder Abuse (to learn about how other countries approach the issue): www.inpea.net

Conclusion

This book has examined some essential issues in community care for health and social care practitioners, students and the general reader. It has focused on carers, the shifting boundaries of community care, care management and assessment, interprofessional working, social support, empowerment, and abuse. Practitioners need to have a sound background knowledge of these topics if they are to develop good, reflective practice. This book has endeavoured to provide this and to make these 'essentials' relevant and comprehensible.

In addition to the topics listed at the start of each chapter, other themes have run throughout the book. This conclusion will summarise these and make some brief comments on developments at the time of writing in early 2006.

First, the book emphasises the importance of bringing the community back into community care. Many of the developments during the 1990s were individualising: assessments, care management, care packages and eligibility criteria all focused on the individual. The book has attempted to balance this by emphasising collectivities of carers and users in a community context.

Second, and this is linked to the previous point, individual problems need to be understood within wider societal structures. Poverty and social divisions such as race, class, gender, age, sexual orientation and disability are key variables in determining people's experiences of community care. Practice needs to be seen within the context of these divisions and inequalities.

Third, there is a need to draw on the strengths of both the formal and the informal sector in order to advance community care. The theme of 'interweaving' or 'partnership' ran through Chapters 2, 4, 5 and 6 in particular. Practitioners need to work effectively with carers and with workers from other agencies and disciplines.

Fourth, 'care' within community care has a 'control' dimension. Chapter 5 noted how this may be true for those people with mental health problems who may be a danger to themselves or others. Chapter 8 discussed the complex issue of adult abuse and the need for a variety of strategies to deal with the problem.

Fifth, the matter of 'shifting boundaries' was introduced in Chapter 3. Community care is rife with boundary, demarcation and funding disputes. This is partially responsible for the 'maze' that the community care system can appear to be to service users and carers.

Sixth, empowerment was a particular theme of Chapter 7 but it also figured in several other chapters. It has been stressed however that real 'democratic' empowerment is difficult to attain.

Finally, the book has discussed some of the contradictions experienced by practitioners in the community care system. Chapter 4 particularly indicated how practitioners may be expected, for example, to undertake individual needs-led assessments in the face of tight resource constraints. This problem is exacerbated by the fact that they are also expected to promote empowerment, anti-oppressive practice and user involvement. There are pressures to meet quality criteria and the demands of computer systems while also being sensitive to the human dilemmas confronting them. There are real contradictions here. The book has tried to make these contradictions more explicit so that practitioners can be aware of the situation they are in and maximise the possibility of constructive change. By making the contradictions explicit, it becomes possible to identify the issues and reflect on a possible way forward. There is a danger of resolving the contradictory expectations by neglecting the real interests of service users. One possibility is to use some of the current rhetoric and guidance on empowerment to try to work out strategies to meet the needs of service users.

After its election in 1997, the Labour government did not set out to restructure the community care system it had inherited. Instead, there have been shifts of emphasis and incremental change over the years. There has been some gradual movement away from the narrow New Right philosophy of the 1980s and the 1990s with its strongly individualistic orientation. With devolution, these changes have varied in their pace and content.

We have noted how devolution has seen differences emerge in the different parts of the United Kingdom. England has seen a division of social services with children's services moving to education and adult services usually remaining as separate departments. This division is not planned for the rest of the UK. A review of social work in Scotland (Scottish Executive, 2006) indicated changes for the future but not a splitting up of the departments.

In all parts of the United Kingdom, there have been strong initiatives to promote interprofessional working. Achieving 'integrated care' is frequently the language used in relation to this. 'Partnership' has been another word used to describe and to indicate this theme of policy. In Scotland, the theme of partnership has perhaps been stronger and more long-lasting with its 'joint futures' agenda. Into the new century in England, a key theme in relation to health and social care has been 'choice', reflected in social care particularly in the promotion of direct payments and individual budgets.

Community care is intrinsically very interesting in terms of social policy and there are some real challenges for the future – most notably in terms of providing appropriately for or an ageing population (Wanless, 2006). Among some interesting changes in the years ahead I would particularly select:

- Developments in 'extra care' housing to enable people to stay in the community but with appropriate support built in.
- The developing use of technology ('telecare') to enable people to live longer and more safely in the community.
- How personal care will be paid for with comparisons of the Scottish 'free' care with the 'means-tested' care in the rest of the United Kingdom?
- How will direct payments develop and what will 'individual budgets' look like?
- Will the single assessment process prove to be helpful or throw up other new problems?

Returning to practice, I have frequently felt humbled by the commitment and caring provided by relatives, friends and neighbours. Equally the attitudes, values and humour of staff have also almost always been impressive. There are a lot of committed and dedicated staff in health and social care who do their very best to help service users and their families through the maze of community care and deal with their issues and problems with genuine sensitivity. It is easy to criticise structures; however a very real positive change has taken place in that there is a more flexible service than there used to be. Although there is much to do, more people can stay at home if they wish to or choose from the more varied housing options.

We have noted how the private sector is now running significant parts of the healthcare and social care systems and I have raised questions about this. There is a daunting amount of form-filling and I have also been surprised at the amount of time spent on computers. However, the dilemmas, problems and crises of service users continue to exist and they require an appropriate human response. There remains then the need for knowledgeable, thoughtful practitioners who will use their skills to try to make the system work for service users and continue to raise questions when services are lacking.

Practitioners and service users know at first hand how well community care provision operates in some respects and how badly in others. Both groups need to exert a strong voice in determining the way forward.

Bibliography

Action on Elder Abuse (AEA) (2004) *Hidden Voices: Older People's Experience of Abuse* (London: Help the Aged).

Age Concern (1986) *The Law and Vulnerable People* (London: Age Concern).

Ahmad, W. I. U. (1996) 'Family Obligations and Social Change Among Asian Communities', in Ahmad, W. I. U. and Atkin, K. (eds) *Race and Community Care* (Buckingham: Open University Press).

Ahmad, W. I. U. and Atkin, K. (eds) (1996) *Race and Community Care* (Buckingham: Open University Press).

Aitken, L. and Griffin, G. (1996) *Gender Issues in Elder Abuse* (London: Sage).

Allen, I. and Perkins, E. (1995) *The Future of Family Care* (London: HMSO).

Ambache, J. (1997) 'Vulnerability and Public Responses', in Decalmer, P. and Glendenning, F. (eds) *The Mistreatment of Elderly People*, 2nd edn (London: Sage).

Arber, S. and Ginn, J. (1991) *Gender and Later Life: A Sociological Analysis of Resources and Constraints* (London: Sage).

Arber, S. and Ginn, J. (1995) 'Gender Differences in Informal Caring', *Health and Social Care in the Community*, 3(1).

Arksey, H. (2002) 'Rationed Care: Assessing the Support Needs of Informal Carers in English Social Services Authorities', *Journal of Social Policy*, 31(1) 81–101.

Atkin, K. and Rollings J. (1993) *Community Care in a Multi-Racial Britain: A Critical Review of the Literature* (London: HMSO).

Atkin, K. and Rollings, J. (1996) 'Looking After Their Own? Family Care-Giving Among Asian and Afro-Caribbean Communities', in Ahmad, W. I. U. and Atkin, K. (eds) *Race and Community Care* (Buckingham: Open University Press).

Attneave, C. (1969) 'Therapy in Tribal Settings and Urban Network Intervention', *Family Process*, 8, 182–210.

Audit Commission (1986) *Making a Reality of Community Care* (London: HMSO).

Audit Commission (1993) *Taking Care* (London: HMSO).

Audit Commission (1994) *Finding a Place: A Review of Mental Health Services For Adults* (London: HMSO).

Audit Commission (1996) *Balancing the Care Equation: Progress with Community Care*, (Community Case Bulletin No 3) (London: Audit Commission).

Audit Commission (1997) *The Coming of Age: Improving Care Services for Older People* (London: Audit Commission).

Audit Commission (1999) *First Assessment* (London: Audit Commission).

Barnes, M. (1997) *Care, Communities and Citizens* (Harlow: Longman).

Barnes, J. A. (1954) 'Class and Committees in a Norwegian Island Parish', *Human Relations*, 7, 39–58.

Barnes, M. and Warren, L. (1999) *Paths to Empowerment* (Bristol: Policy Press).

Barr, A., Drysdale, J. and Henderson, P. (1997) *Towards Caring Communities* (Brighton: Pavilion).

Barr, A., Stenhouse, C. and Henderson, P. (2001) *Caring Communities* (York: Joseph Rowntree Foundation).

Bass, M. and Drewett, R. (1997) *Real Work: Supported Employment for People With Learning Difficulties* (Sheffield: Joint Unit for Social Services Research).

Bayley, J. (1998) *Iris: A Memoir of Iris Murdoch* (London: Duckworth).

Bayley, M. (1973) *Mental Handicap and Community Care* (London: Routledge and Kegan Paul).

Bennett, G., Kingston, P. and Penhale, B. (1997) *The Dimensions of Elder Abuse* (London: Macmillan).

Beresford, P. (1997) 'The Last Social Division? Revisiting the Relationship Between Social Policy, its Producers and Consumers', in May, M., Brunsdon, E. and Craig, G. (eds), *Social Policy Review 9* (London: Social Policy Association).

Beresford, P. and Croft, S. (1993) *Citizen Involvement* (London: Macmillan).

Biegel, D. E., Shore, B. K. and Gordon, E. (1984) *Building Support Networks for the Elderly* (London: Sage).

Biggs, S. (1996) 'A Family Concern: Elder Abuse in British Social Policy', *Critical Social Policy*, 16(2).

Biggs, S., Phillipson, C. and Kingston, P. (eds) (1995) *Elder Abuse in Perspective* (Buckingham: Open University Press).

Bott, E. (1957) *Family and Social Network* (London: Tavistock).

Brammer, A. (1996) 'Elder Abuse in the UK: A New Jurisdiction?', *Journal of Elder Abuse & Neglect*, 8(2).

Brandon, D. (1995) *Advocacy* (Birmingham: Venture).

Brown, H. C. (1998) *Social Work and Sexuality* (London: Macmillan).

Brown, H. and Smith, H. (1992) *Normalisation* (London: Routledge).

Bulmer, M. (1987) *The Social Basis of Community Care* (London: Allen and Unwin).

Bunting M. (2004) *The Hidden Toll We All Pay* (Guardian, 21 June: London).

Burns, D. and Taylor, M. (1998) *Mutual Aid and Self-Help* (Bristol: Policy Press).

Butler, R. (1987) 'Agism', in *Encyclopaedia of Aging* (New York: Springer).

Bytheway, B., Bacigalupo, V., Bornat, J., Johnson, J. and Spur, S. (2002) *Understanding Care, Welfare and Community; A Reader* (Routledge, London).

Campbell, J. and Oliver, M. (1996) *Disability Politics* (London: Routledge).

Caplan, G. (1974a) 'Support Systems', in Caplan, G. (ed.) *Support Systems and Community Mental Health* (New York: Basic Books).

Caplan, G. (ed.) (1974b) *Support Systems and Community Mental Health* (New York: Basic Books).

Carers UK (2002) *Without U...? Calculating the value of carers' support* (London; Carers UK).

Carers UK (2005) *Facts About Carers* (London; Carers UK).

Carpenter, J., Schneider, J., Brandon, T. and Wooff, D. (2003) 'Working in Multidisciplinary Mental Health Teams: The Impact on Social Workers and Health Professionals of Integrated Mental Health Care', *British Journal of Social Work*, 33, 1081–1103.

Carter, T. and Beresford, P. (2000) *Age and Change* (York: Joseph Rowntree Foundation).

Cassel, J. (1974) 'Psychosocial Processes and Stress: Theoretical Formulations' *International Journal of Health Services*, 4, 471–82.

Challis, D. (1999) 'Assessment and Care Management: Developments since the Community Care Reforms', in Sutherland, S. R. (Royal Commission on Long Term Care), *Research Vol. 3* (London: Stationery Office).

Child Poverty Action Group (2005) *Paying for Care Handbook*, 5th edn (London: CPAG).

CI(92)34 (1992) Letter from Herbert Laming (chief social services inspector) on assessment, 14 December (London: DoH).

Clarke, S. (1998) 'Community Development and Health Professionals', in Symonds, A. and Kelly, A. (eds) *The Social Construction of Community Care* (London: Macmillan).

Clements, L. (2004) *Community Care and the Law*, 3rd edn (London: Legal Action Group).

Clough, R. (1996) *The Abuse of Adults in Residential Institutions* (London: Whiting & Birch).

Cobb, S. (1976) 'Social Support as a Moderator of Life Stress', *Psychosomatic Medicine*, 38, 300–314.

Cohen, S. and Syme, S. L. (1985) *Social Support and Health* (London: Academic Press).

Collins, A. H. and Pancoast, D. L. (1976) *Natural Helping Networks* (Washington: National Association of Social Workers).

Commission for Social Care Inspection (2004) *Leaving Hospital – the price of delays* (London: CSCI).

Commission for Social Care Inspection (2005) *Leaving Hospital – revisited* (London: CSCI).

Cooper, H., Arber, S., Fee, L. and Ginn, J. (1999) *The Influence of Social Support and Social Capital on Health* (London: HEA).

Cormie, J. (1999) 'The Fife User Panels Project: Empowering Older People', in Barnes, M. and Warren, L. (eds) *Paths to Empowerment* (Bristol: Policy Press).

Craft, A. (1996) 'Abuse of Younger and Older People: Similarities and Difference', in Clough, R., *The Abuse of Adults in Residential Institutions* (London: Whiting & Birch).

Crewe, N. M. and Zola, I. K. (1983) *Independent Living for Physically Disabled People* (London: Jossey-Bass).

Croft, S. and Beresford, P. (1999) 'Elder Abuse and Participation: A Crucial Coupling for Change', in Slater, P. and Eastman, M. (eds) *Elder Abuse* (London: Age Concern).

CSCI (2004) *Direct Payments: What are the barriers?* (London: CSCI).

Dalley, G. (1989) 'Professional Ideology or Organisational Tribalism?', in Taylor, R. and Ford, J. (eds) *Social Work and Health Care* (London: Jessica Kingsley).

Dalley, G. (1996) *Ideologies of Caring*, 2nd edn (London: Macmillan).

Davey, B. (1999) 'Solving Economic, Social and Environmental Problems Together: An Empowerment Strategy for Losers', in Barnes, M. and Warren, L. (eds) *Paths To Empowerment* (Bristol: Policy Press).

Davies, L. and Leonard, P. (2004) *Social Work in a Corporate Era* (Aldershot: Ashgate).

Davis, A., Ellis, K. and Rummery, K. (1997) *Access to Assessment* (Bristol: Policy Press).

Dearden, C. and Becker, S. (2004) *Young Carers in the UK: The 2004 Report* (London: Carers UK).

DHSS (1981) *Growing Older* (London: HMSO).

DHSS (Northern Ireland) (1990) *People First: Community Care in Northern Ireland* (Belfast: HMSO).

Dobash, R. E. and Dobash, R. (1992) *Women, Violence and Social Change* (London: Routledge).

DoH (1989a) *Caring for People* (London: HMSO).

DoH (1989b) *Working for Patients* (London: HMSO).

DoH (1990) *Community Care in the Next Decade and Beyond: Policy Guidance* (London: HMSO).

DoH (1991a) *Care Management and Assessment: Managers' Guide* (London: HMSO).

DoH (1991b) *Care Management and Assessment: Practitioners' Guide* (London: HMSO).

DoH (1993) *No Longer Afraid: Practice Guidelines* (London: HMSO).

DoH (1994) *Key Area Handbook: Mental Illness*, 2nd edn (London: HMSO).

DoH (1995a) *Building Bridges* (London: DoH).

DoH (1995b) *Practical Guidance on Joint Commissioning for Project Leaders* (London: DoH).

DoH (1997a) *The New NHS: Modern, Dependable* (London: HMSO).

DoH (1998a) *Modernising Social Services* (London: DoH).

DoH (1998b) *They Look After Their Own, Don't They?* (London: DoH).

DoH (1998c) *Modernising Mental Health Services* (London: DoH).

DoH (1998d) *Partnership in Action* (London: DoH).

DoH (1999a) *Caring About Carers* (London: DoH).

DoH (1999b) *Saving Lives: Our Healthier Nation* (London: DoH).

DoH (2000a) *No Secrets: Guidance on Developing Multi-Agency Policies and Procedures to Protect Vulnerable Adults from Abuse* (London: HMSO).

DoH (2000b) *The NHS Plan. A Plan for Investment, a Plan for Reform*, CM 4818-1 (London: HMSO).

DoH (2001a) *A Practitioner's Guide to Assessment under the Carers and Disabled Children Act 2000* (London: DoH).

DoH (2001b) *Valuing People: A New Strategy for Learning Disability for the 21st Century* (London: HMSO).

DoH (2001c) *National Service Framework for Older People* (London: DoH).

DoH (2002a) *Planning With People: Towards Person Centred Approaches: Guidance for Implementation Groups* (London: HMSO).

DoH (2002b) *Planning With People: Towards Person Centred Approaches: Guidance for Partnership Boards* (London: HMSO).

DoH (2002c) *Mental Health Implementation Guide: Community Mental Health Teams* (London: HMSO).

DoH (2002d) *Fair Access to Care Services: Guidance on Eligibility Criteria for Adult Social Care* (London: DoH).

DoH (2004a) *The NHS Improvement Plan – Putting People at the Heart of Public Services* Department of Health, CM 6268 (London: TSO).

DoH (2004b) *Choosing Health: Making Healthy Choices Easier* (London: DoH).

DoH (2005a) *Delivering race equality in mental health care and The Government's response to the independent inquiry into the death of David Bennett* (London: DoH).

DoH (2005b) *Independence, Well-being and Choice* (London: DoH).

DoH (2005c) *Carers and Disabled Children Act 2000 and Carers (Equal Opportunities) Act 2004 Combined Policy Guidance* (London: DoH).

DoH (2006) *Our Health, Our Care, Our Say: A New Direction for Community Services* (London: DoH).

Douglas, A. and Philpot, T. (1998) *Caring and Coping* (London: Routledge).

Dowling, B., Powell, M. and Glendinning C. (2004) 'Conceptualising Successful Partnerships', *Health and Social Care in the Community*, 12(4), 309–17.

Eastman, M. (1984) *Old Age Abuse* (Mitcham: Age Concern).

Eastman, M. (1994) *Old Age Abuse* (London: Chapman & Hall/Age Concern).

Eastman, M. (1999) 'Elder Abuse and Professional Intervention: A Social Welfare Model?', in Slater, P. and Eastman, M. (eds) *Elder Abuse* (London: Age Concern).

Eley, S. (2003) 'Diversity Among Carers', in Stalker, K. (ed.) *Reconceptualising Work With 'Carers'* (London: Jessica Kingsley).

Ell, K. (1996) 'Social Networks, Social Support and Coping with Serious Illness: The Family Connection', *Social Science and Medicine*, 42(2), 173–83.

Ellis, K. (1993) *Squaring the Circle* (York: Joseph Rowntree Foundation).

Family Policy Studies Centre (1997) *A Guide to Family Issues: Family Briefing Paper 2* (London: Family Policy Studies Centre).

Field J. (2003) *Social Capital* (London: Routledge).

Finch, J. (1989) *Family Obligations and Social Change* (Cambridge: Polity Press).

Finch J. (1995) 'Responsibilities, Obligations and Commitments', in Allen, I. and Perkins, E. (eds) *The Future of Family Care* (London: HMSO).

Finch, J. and Groves, D. (eds) (1983) *A Labour of Love: Women, Work and Caring* (London: RKP).

Finch, J. and Mason, J. (1993) *Negotiating Family Responsibilities* (London: Routledge).

Firth, P., Luff, G. and D. Oliviere (eds) (2005) *Loss, Change and Bereavement in Palliative Care* (London: Open University Press).

Fischer, C. (1982) *To Dwell among Friends* (Chicago, IL.: University of Chicago Press).

Fook, J. (2002) *Social Work: Critical Theory and Practice* (London: Sage).

Freire, P. (1972) *Pedagogy of the Oppressed* (London: Penguin).

Friedman, S. R. (1999) *Social Networks, Drug Injectors' Lives and HIV/AIDS* (London: Plenum).

Froland, C., Pancoast, D. L., Chapman, N. J. and Kimboko, P. J. (1981) *Helping Networks and Human Services* (Beverly Hills, CA: Sage).

Galanter (1999) *Network Therapy for Alcohol and Drug Abuse* (New York: Guilford Press).

Galvin, S. W. and McCarthy, S. (1994) 'Multi-Disciplinary Community Team: Clinging to the Wreckage', *Journal of Mental Health*, 3, 157–66.

Glasby, J. (2003) *Hospital Discharge* (Oxford: Radcliffe Medical Press).

Glasby, J. and Littlechild, R. (2004) *The Health and Social Care Divide* (Bristol: Policy Press).

Glasby, J. Littlechild, R. and Price, K. (2004) 'Show Me the Way to go Home: A Narrative Review of the Literature on Delayed Hospital Discharges and Older People', *British Journal of Social Work*, 34, 1189–97.

Glendinning, C. Halliwell, S. Jacobs, S. Rummery, K. and Tyrer, J. (2000) *Buying Independence* (Bristol: Policy Press).

Gottlieb, B. H. (1983) *Social Support Strategies* (Thousand Oaks, CA: Sage).

Grant, L. (1999) *Remind Me Who I Am, Again* (London: Granta).

Green, H. (1988) *Informal Carers* (London: HMSO).

Griffiths, R. (1988) *Community Care: Agenda for Action* (London: HMSO).

Griffiths, D. Sigona, N. and Zetter, R. (2005) *Refugee Community Organisations and Dispersal* (Bristol: Policy Press).

Hadley, R. and Clough, R. (1996) *Care in Chaos* (London: Cassell).

Halpern, D. (2005) *Social Capital* (Cambridge: Polity Press).

Hancock, M. and Villeneau, R. (1997) *Effective Partnerships* (London: Sainsbury Centre).

Harding, T., Meredith, B. and Wistow, G. (1996) *Options for Long-Term Care* (London: HMSO).

Harris, J. (2003) *The Social Work Business* (London: Routledge).

Hasler, F. and Stewart, A. (2004) *Making Direct Payments Work: identifying and overcoming the barriers to implementation* (Brighton: Pavilion).

Health Service Commissioner (1994) *Failure to Provide Long-Term NHS Care for a Brain-Damaged Patient* HC197 (London: HMSO).

Heron, C. (1998) *Working with Carers* (London: Jessica Kingsley).

Hill, M. (2002) 'Network Assessments and Diagrams: A Flexible Friend for Social Work Practice and Education', *Journal of Social Work*, 2(2), 233–54.

Hillery, G. A. (1955) 'Definitions of Community: Areas of Agreement' *Rural Sociology* 50, 20–35.

Hills, J. (2002) 'Does a Focus on "Social Exclusion" Change the Policy Response?' in Hills, J. Le Grand, J. and Piachaud, D. (eds) *Understanding Social Exclusion* (Oxford: Oxford University Press).

Holman, B. (1993) *A New Deal for Social Welfare* (Oxford: Lion Publishing).

House of Commons Health Committee (HoC) (1995) *Long-Term Care: NHS Responsibilities for Meeting Continuing Health Care Needs* first report, vols 1–3 (London: HMSO).

House of Commons Health Committee (HoC) (1999) *The Relationship between Health and Social Services*, Vol. 1 (London: Stationery Office).

House of Commons Health Committee (HoC) (2002) *Delayed Discharges (third report)* (London: Stationery Office).

House of Commons Health Committee (HoC) (2004) *Elder Abuse: Second Report of Session 2003–04*, Vol. 1 (London: Stationery Office).

Hudson B. (2005) 'Pick up the Pieces', *Community Care*, 22–28 September, pp. 36–7.

Jack, R. (1995) *Empowerment in Community Care* (London: Chapman & Hall).

Katbamna, S., Ahmad, W., Bhakta, P., and Parker, G. (2004) 'Do they look after their own? Informal support for South Asian carers', *Health and Social Care in the Community*, 12(5), 398–406.

Kawachi, I. and Berkman, L. (2001) Social Ties and Mental Health, *Journal of Urban Health*, 78(3), 458–65.

King's Fund Centre (1991) *Meeting the Challenge* (London: King Edward's Hospital Fund).

Kingston, P. and Penhale, B. (eds) (1995) *Family Violence and the Caring Professions* (London: Macmillan).

Kubler-Ross, E. (1969) *On Death and Dying* (New York: Macmillan).

LAC(92)27 (1992) National Assistance Act (1948) *Choice of Accommodation Directions* (London: DoH).

LAC(93)4 (1993) *Community Care Plans (Consultation) Directions* (London: DoH).

LAC(95)5 (1995) *NHS Responsibilities for Meeting Continuing Health Care Needs* (London: DoH).

LAC(97)15 (1997) *Family Law Act (1996 Part 1V, Family Homes and Domestic Violence, Responsibilities of Local Authorities and the Guardian Ad Litem and Reporting Officer Service* (London: DoH).

LAC(2001)18 (2001) *Continuing care: NHS and local councils' responsibilities* (London: DoH).

Law Commission (1995) *Mental Incapacity* (London: HMSO).

Lawson, J. (1999) 'Developing a Policy on Abuse in Residential and Nursing Homes', in Pritchard, J. (ed.) *Elder Abuse Work* (London: Jessica Kingsley).

Learning Disability Advisory Group (2000) *Fulfilling the Promises: Proposals for a Framework for Services for People with Learning Disabilities* (Learning Disability Advisory Group: www.wales.gov.uk).

Leason, K. (2005) 'Curtains for Care Homes', *Community Care*, 7–11 April.

Leathard, A. (1997) 'The New Boundaries of Health and Welfare in Collaborative Care', in May, M., Brunsdon, E. and Craig, G., *Social Policy Review 9* (London: Social Policy Association).

Leathard, A. (ed.) 2003 *Interprofessional Collaboration* (Hove: Brunner-Routledge).

Leece, J. (2004), 'Money Talks, but What Does it Say? Direct Payments and the Commodification of Care', *Practice*, 16(3), 211–21.

Lewis, J. and Glennerster, H. (1996) *Implementing the New Community Care* (Buckingham: Open University Press).

Lewis, J. and Meredith, B. (1988) *Daughters Who Care: Daughters Caring for Mothers at Home* (London: RKP).

Lipsky, M. (1980) *Street Level Bureaucracy: Dilemmas of the Individual in Public Services* (New York: Russell Sage Foundation).

Litwin, H. (1995) *Uprooted in Old Age* (Westport: Greenwood Press).

Litwin, H. (1997) 'Social Network Type and Health Service Utilization', *Research on Aging*, 19(3), 274–99.

Litwin, H. (1998) 'Social Network Type and Health Status in a National Sample of Elderly Israelis', *Social Science and Medicine*, 46(4–5), 599–609.

Litwin, H. (1999) 'Support Network Type and Patterns of Help Giving and Receiving Among Older Adults', *Journal of Social Service Research*, 24(3–4), 83–101.

Local Government Association (LGA) (1997) *Removing the Barriers: The Case for a New Deal for Social Services and Social Security* (London: LGA).

Lord Chancellor's Department (1997) *Who Decides?* (London: HMSO).

Loxley, A. (1997) *Collaboration in Health and Welfare* (London: Jessica Kingsley).

Mandelstam, M. (2005) *Community Care Practice and the Law*, 3rd edn (London: Jessica Kingsley).

Mansell, J. and Beadle-Brown, J. (2004) 'Person Centred Planning or Person Centred Action? Policy and Practice in Intellectual Disability Services', *Journal of Applied Research in Intellectual Disabilities*, 17(1), 1–9.

Manthorpe, J. (1999) 'Putting Elder Abuse on the Agenda: Achievements of a Campaign', in Slater, P. and Eastman, M. (eds) *Elder Abuse* (London: Age Concern).

Manthorpe, J. (2003) 'Nearest and Dearest? The Neglect of Lesbians in Caring Relationships', *British Journal of Social Work*, 33(6), 753–68.

May, M., Brunsdon, E. and Craig, G. (1997) *Social Policy Review 9* (London: Social Policy Association).

Mayo, M. (1998) 'Community Work', in Adams, R., Dominelli, L. and Payne, M. (eds) *Social Work: Themes, Issues and Critical Debates* (London: Macmillan).

McCreadie, C. (1994) 'Introduction: The Issues, Practice and Policy', in Eastman, M. (ed.) *Old Age Abuse* (London: Chapman & Hall).

McCreadie, C. (1996) *Elder Abuse: Update on Research* (London: Institute of Gerontology).

Means, R., Richards, S. and Smith, R. (2003) *Community Care: Policy and Practice*, 3rd edn (London: Palgrave Macmillan).

Mencap (1999) *Fully Charged* (London: Mencap).

Mills, C. W. (1959) *The Sociological Imagination* (Oxford: Oxford University Press).

Milner, J. and O'Byrne, P. (2002) *Assessment in Social Work*, 2nd edn (Basingstoke: Palgrave).

Morgan, S. (2000) *Clinical Risk Management: A Clinical Tool and Practitioner Manual* (London: Sainsbury Centre for Mental Health).

Morris, J. (1993) *Independent Lives* (London: Macmillan).

National Assembly for Wales (2000a) *In Safe Hands* (Wales: Social Services Inspectorate).

National Assembly for Wales (2000b) *Caring About Carers: A Srategy for Carers in Wales. Implementation Plan* (Cardiff: National Assembly for Wales).

NHSE/SSI (1999) *Effective Care Coordination In Mental Health Services: Modernising the care programme approach* (DH 16736).

National Institute for Mental Health (2003) *Inside Outside – Improving Mental Health Services for Black and Minority Ethnic Communities in England* (London: DoH).

Nocon, A. and Baldwin, S. (1998) *Trends in Rehabilitation Policy* (London: King's Fund).

Nolan, M., Grant, G. and Keady, J. (1996) *Understanding Family Care* (Buckingham: Open University Press).

Nolan, M., Lundh, U. Grant, G. and Keady, J. (2003) *Partnerships in Family Care* (Buckingham: Open University Press).

Norfolk, Suffolk and Cambridgeshire Strategic Health Authority (2003) *Independent Inquiry into the Death of David Bennett* Cambridge.

North, C., Ritchie, J. and Ward, K. (1993) *Factors Influencing the Implementation of the Care Programme Approach* (London: HMSO).

Ogg, J. and Bennett, G. (1992) 'Elder Abuse in Britain', *British Medical Journal*, 305, 998–9.

Oldman, C. (2003) 'Deceiving, theorizing and self-justification: a critique of independent living', *Critical Social Policy*, 23(1), 44–62.

Oliver, M. (1990) *The Politics of Disablement* (London: Macmillan).

Oliver, M. (1996) *Understanding Disability: From Theory to Practice* (Basingstoke: Macmillan).

Oliver, M. and Sapey, B. (2006) *Social Work with Disabled People*, 3rd Edn (Basingstoke: Palgrave Macmillan).

Onyett, S. (1997) 'Collaboration and the Community Health Team', *Journal of Interprofessional Care*, 11(3).

Onyett, S. (2003) *Teamworking in Mental Health* (Basingstoke: Palgrave).

Onyett, S. and Ford, R. (1996) 'Multidisciplinary Community Teams: Where is the Wreckage', *Journal of Mental Health*, 5(1), 47–55.

Onyett, S., Heppleston, T. and Bushnell, D. (1994) 'A National Survey of Community Mental Health Teams', *Journal of Mental Health*, 3, 175–94.

Onyett, S., Pillinger, T. and Muijen, M. (1995) *Making Community Mental Health Teams Work* (London: Sainsbury Centre for Mental Health).

Parker, G. and Lawton, D. (1994) *Different Types of Care, Different Types of Carer: Evidence from the General Household Survey* (London: HMSO).

Parkinson, M. (1998) *Combating Social Exclusion* (Bristol: Policy Press).

Parsloe, P. (ed.) (1999) *Risk Assessment in Social Care and Social Work* (London: Jessica Kingsley).

Parton, N. (2004) 'Post-Theories for Practice: Challenging the Dogmas', in Davies, L. and Leonard, P. (eds) *Social Work in a Corporate Era* (Aldershot: Ashgate).

Parton, N. and O'Byrne, P. (2000) *Constructive Social Work: Towards a New Practice* (Basingstoke: Palgrave).

Patmore, C. and Weaver, T. (1991) *Community Mental Health Teams: Lessons for Planners and Managers* (London: Good Practices in Mental Health).

Payne, M. (1995) *Social Work and Community Care* (London: Macmillan).

Pease, B. and Fook, J. (1999) *Transforming Social Work Practice* (London: Routledge).

Penhale, B. and Kingston, P. (1995) 'Social Perspectives on Elder Abuse', in Kingston, P. and Penhale, B. (eds) *Family Violence and the Caring Professions* (London: Macmillan).

Perry J. (2004) 'Hate Crime Against People With Learning Disabilities', *Journal of Adult Protection*, 6(1).

Petch, A. (2003) *Intermediate Care* (York: Joseph Rowntree Foundation).

Petch, A., Cheetham, J., Fuller, R., MacDonald, C. and Myers, F. (1996) *Delivering Community Care* (Edinburgh: Stationery Office).

Phillipson, C., Allan, G. and Morgan, D. (2004) *Social Networks and Social Exclusion* (Aldershot: Ashgate).

Pillemer, K. A. and Wolf, R. (eds) (1986) *Elder Abuse: Conflict in the Family* (New York: Auburn House).

Pollock, A. (2004) *NHS plc: The Privatisation of Our Health Service* (London: Verso).

Poxton, R. (1996) 'Bridging the Gap: Joint Commissioning of Health and Social Care', in Harrison, A. (ed.) *Health Care UK 1995–1996* (London: King's Fund).

Priestley, M. (1999) *Disability Politics and Community Care* (London: Jessica Kingsley).

Prime Minister's Strategy Unit (2005) *Improving the Life Chances of Disabled People* (London, Cabinet Office).

Pritchard, J. (1995) *The Abuse of Older People*, 2nd edn (London: Jessica Kingsley).

Pritchard, J. (1996) *Working with Elder Abuse: A Training Manual for Home Care Residential and Day Care Staff* (London: Jessica Kingsley).

Putnam, R. D. (2000) *Bowling Alone: the collapse and revival of American community* (New York: Simon & Schuster).

Quinn, A. (2005) 'The context of loss, change and bereavement in palliative care', in P. Firth, G. Luff and D. Oliviere (eds) *Loss, Change and Bereavement in Palliative Care* (London: Open University Press).

Qureshi, H. and Walker, A. (1989) *The Caring Relationship* (London: Macmillan).

Richards, S. (2000) 'Bridging the Divide: Elders and the Assessment Process', *British Journal of Social Work*, 30, 37–49.

Ritchie, J., Dick, D. and Lingham, R. (1994) *The Report of the Inquiry into the Care and Treatment of Christopher Clunis* (London: HMSO).

Ritchie, P., Sanderson, H., Kilbane, J., Routledge, M. (2003) *People Plans and Practicalities: Achieving Change Through Person Centred Planning* (Edinburgh: SHS Trust).

Robb, B. (1967) *Sans Everything: A Case to Answer* (London: Thomas Nelson).

Robson, P., Locke, M. and Dawson, J. (1997) *Consumerism or Democracy* (Bristol: Policy Press).

Rueveni, U. (1979) *Networking Families in Crisis* (New York: Human Sciences Press).

Scottish Executive (1999a) *The Strategy for Carers in Scotland* (Edinburgh: Scottish Executive).

Scottish Executive (1999b) *The Same as You? A Review of Services for People with Learning Disabilities* (Edinburgh: Scottish Executive).

Scottish Executive (2005) *Better Outcomes for Older People: Framework for Joint Services* (Edinburgh: Scottish Executive).

Scottish Executive (2006) *Changing Lives* (Edinburgh: Scottish Executive).

Scourfield, P. (2005) 'Implementing the Community Care (Direct Payments) Act: Will the Supply of Personal Assistants meet the Demand and at what Price?', *Journal of Social Policy*, 34(3), 469–88.

Sharkey, P. J. (1989) 'Social Networks and Social Service Workers', *British Journal of Social Work*, 19, 387–405.

Sharkey, P. J. (1995) *Introducing Community Care* (London: Collins Educational).

Sharkey, P. J. (2000a) 'Community Work and Community Care: Links in Practice and in Education' *Social Work Education*, 19(1), 7–17.

Sharkey, P. J. (2000b) 'Community Care, Community Work and Social Exclusion', in Paylor, I., Froggett L. and Harris, J. (eds) *Reclaiming Social Work: The Southport Papers Volume Two* (Birmingham: BASW).

Sheppard, M. (1995) *Care Management and the New Social Work* (London: Whiting and Birch).

Silverman, P. R. (2005) 'Mourning: a changing view', in P. Firth, G. Luff and D. Oliviere (eds) (2005) *Loss, Change and Bereavement in Palliative Care* (London: Open University Press).

Simpson, A., Miller, C. and Bowers, L. (2003) 'The history of the Care Programme Approach in England: Where did it go wrong?' *Journal of Mental Health*, 12(5), 489–504.

Slater, P. (1999) 'Elder Abuse as Harm to Older Adults: The Relevance of Age', in Slater, P. and Eastman, M. (eds) *Elder Abuse* (London: Age Concern).

Slater, P. and Eastman, M. (1999) (eds) *Elder Abuse* (London: Age Concern).

Smale, G., Tuson, G., Biehal, N. and Marsh, P. (1993) *Empowerment, Assessment, Care Management and the Skilled Worker* (London: HMSO).

Smale, G., Tuson, G. and Statham, D. (2000) *Social Work and Social Problems* (Basingstoke: Macmillan).

Small, N. and Rhodes, P. (2000) *Too Ill To Talk* (London, Routledge).

Social Exclusion Unit (SEU) (1998) *Bringing Britain Together: A National Strategy for Neighbourhood Renewal* (London: HMSO).

Social Exclusion Unit (SEU) (2004a) *Mental Health and Social Exclusion* (London: ODPM).

Social Exclusion Unit (SEU) (2004b) *The Impact of Government Policy on Social Exclusion Among Older People* (London: ODPM).

Social Exclusion Unit (SEU) (2006) *A Sure Start to Later Life: Ending Inequalities for Older People* (London: ODPM).

Spandler, H. (2004) 'Friend or Foe? Towards a Critical Assessment of Direct Payments', *Critical Social Policy*, 24(2), 187–209.

Speck, R. and Attneave, C. (1973) *Family Networks* (New York: Pantheon).

Spokes, J., Pare, M. and Royle G. (1988) *The Report of the Committee of Inquiry into the Care and Aftercare of Miss Sharon Campbell* (London: HMSO).

Stalker, K. (ed.) (2003) *Reconceptualising Work With 'Carers'* (London: Jessica Kingsley).

Stalker, K., Baron, S., Riddell, S. and Wilkinson, H. (1999) 'Models of Disability: The Relationship Between Theory and Practice in Non-Statutory Organisations', *Critical Social Policy*, 19(1).

Stewart, M. J. (1993) *Integrating Social Support and Nursing* (London: Sage).

Stockford, D. (1988) *Integrating Care Systems* (London: Longman).

Stroebe, M. and Schut, H. (1999) 'The Dual Process Model of Coping with Bereavement: Rationale and Description', *Death Studies*, 23, 197–224.

Sutherland, S. R. (Royal Commission on Long Term Care) (1999) *With Respect to Old Age: Long term care – rights and responsibilities: a report* Cm 4192-1 (London: Stationery Office).

Swain, J., French, S., Barnes, C. and Thomas, C. (2004) *Disabling Barriers – Enabling Environments*, 2nd edn (London: Sage).

Szivos, S. (1992) 'The Limits to Integration', in Brown, H. and Smith, H. (eds) *Normalisation* (London: Routledge).

Taylor, R. and Ford, J. (1989) *Social Work and Health Care* (London: Jessica Kingsley).

Taylor, S. (1993) 'Social Integration, Social Support and Health', in Taylor, S. and Field, D. (eds), *Sociology of Health and Health Care* (Oxford: Blackwell).

Thompson, N. (1995) *Age and Dignity* (Aldershot: Arena).

Thompson, N. (2002) (ed.) *Loss and Grief* (London: Palgrave).

Thompson, N. (2003) *Promoting Equality*, 2nd edn (London: Palgrave).

Thompson, N. (2006) *Anti-Discriminatory Practice*, 4th edn (London: Palgrave).

Thompson, P. and Matthews, D. (2004) *Fair Enough* (London: Age Concern England).

Thornton, P. and Tozer, R. (1995) *Having a Say in Change: Older People and Community Care* (York: Joseph Rowntree Foundation).

Titmus, R. (1973) *The Gift Relationship* (London: Penguin).

Townsend, P. (1962) *The Last Refuge* (London: Routledge and Kegan Paul).

Trevillion, S. (1999) *Networking and Community Partnership* (Aldershot: Ashgate).

Trimble, D. and Kliman, J. (1995) in Elkaim, M. (ed.) *Panorama des Therapies Familiales* (Paris: Editions du Seuil).

Truax, C. B. and Carkhuff, R. R. (1967) *Towards Effective Counselling and Psychotherapy: Training and Practice* (New York: Aldine).

Twigg, J. (1989) 'Models of Care: How do Social Care Agencies Conceptualise their Relationship with Informal Carers', *Journal of Social Policy*, 18(1).

Twigg, J. (1992) *Carers; Research and Practice* (London: HMSO).

Twigg, J. and Atkin, K. (1994) *Carers Perceived* (Buckingham: Open University Press).

Ungerson, C. (1987) *Policy is Personal: Sex, Gender and Informal Caring* (London: Tavistock).

Ungerson, C. (2002) 'Care as a commodity', in Bytheway, B., Bacigalupo, V., Bornat, J., Johnson, J. and Spur, S. (2002) *Understanding Care, Welfare and Community; A Reader* (Routledge, London).

Utting, W. (1994) *Creating Community Care* (London: Mental Health Foundation).

Walker, S. and Beckett, C. (2003) *Social Work Assessment and Intervention* (Lyme Regis: Russell House).

Wanless, D. (2006) *Securing Good Care for Older People: Taking a Long-Term View* (London: King's Fund).

Wardhaugh, J. and Wilding, P. (1993) 'Towards an Explanation of the Corruption of Care' *Critical Social Policy*, 47, 4–31.

Weiner, K., Hughes, J., Challis, D. and Pedersen, I. (2003) 'Integrating Health and Social Care at the Micro Level: Health Care Professionals as Care Managers for Older People', *Social Policy & Administration*, 37(5), 498–515.

Wells, J. S. G. (1997) 'Priorities, "Street Level Bureaucracy" and the Community Mental Health Team', *Health and Social Care in the Community*, 5(5), 333–42.

Wenger, G. C. (1984) *The Supportive Network: Coping with Old Age* (London: Allen & Unwin).

Wenger, G. C. (1994) *Support Networks of Older People: A Guide for Practitioners* (Bangor: Centre For Social Policy Research and Development, University of Wales).

Wenger, G. C. and Day, B. (1995) *Support Networks of Older People* (Brighton: Pavilion).

Wenger, G. C. and Tucker, I. (2002) 'Using Network Variations In Practice: Identification of Support Network Type', *Health and Social Care in the Community*, 10(1), 28–33.

Whittaker, T. (1995) 'Violence, Gender and Elder Abuse: Towards a Feminist Analysis and Practice', *Journal of Gender Studies*, 4(1), 35–45.

Whittaker, J. K. and Garbarino, J. (1983) *Social Support Networks* (New York: Aldine de Gruyter).

Wilkinson, R. G. (2005) *The Impact of Inequality: How to Make Sick Societies Healthier* (London: Routledge).

Williams, F. (2001) 'In and beyond New Labour: Towards a new political ethics of care', *Critical Social Policy*, 21(4), 467–93.

Williams, F. (2004a) *Rethinking Families* (London: Caloustie Gulbenkian Foundation).

Williams, L. (2004b) 'Refugees and asylum seekers as a group at risk of adult abuse', *Journal of Adult Protection*, 6(4), 4–15.

Williams, P. and Shoultz, B. (1982) *We Can Speak for Ourselves* (London: Souvenir).

Wistow, G. and Brooks, T. (1988) *Planning and Joint Management* (London: RIPA).

Wistow, G., Knapp, M., Hardy, B., Forder, J., Kendall, J. and Manning, R. (1996) *Social Care Markets* (Buckingham: Open University Press).

Wittenberg, R., Comas-Herrera, A., Pickard, L. and Hancock, R. (2004) *Future Demand For Long-term Care in the UK* (York; Joseph Rowntree Foundation).

Wolfensberger, W. (1972) *The Principle of Normalisation in Human Services* (Toronto: National Institute on Mental Retardation).

Wright, F. (2000) *Capital Offences: Variations in local authority treatment of older home owners entering residential care* (London: Age Concern/Institute of Gerontology).

Index